Advance Praise for *Trying*

"Like a life-changing pair of pants, Chloé Caldwell's *Trying* offered a grip at once intimate and transformative. This book is made of life but also totally *made*, whittled and sculpted with the keen eye of a craftsman, propulsively carried by the quicksilver pivots of feeling and noticing that are Caldwell's great gifts to her readers. *Trying* moved me and consumed me; it's a great gutting swirl of grief and freedom and vitality. A searing whispered vision. I am grateful for it."

—Leslie Jamison, author of *Splinters: Another Kind of Love Story*

"Chloé Caldwell describes desire like no one else. Her writing is honesty as poetry. Every sentence is intimate and stunning, and it will take you weeks from when you arrive at the end of this book to extricate yourself from Caldwell's brain, to separate your thoughts from hers, to even want to. She writes about fear, hope, and disappointment with such self-awareness and empathy that you, too, will want to step out of your comfort zone, acknowledge your truths, and get acquainted with the reasons behind your want. In *Trying*, Caldwell exposes the messiness of growth, forgiveness, and moving on. In doing so, she gives both herself and her readers the permission to consider all possibilities, to keep reimagining our lives until they are finally ours, to try and try again."

—Jill Louise Busby, author of *Unfollow Me: Essays on Complicity*

"In *Trying*, Chloé Caldwell begins and ends alone. A process of creation is thwarted. She repeats the cycle over and over until a rupture ensures it cannot be repeated again. When I finished reading the book, I began it again. I found pleasure in the limbo, in the between. I wanted to be in Chloé's language forever."

—LA Warman, author of *Dust* and *Whore Foods*

"Chloé Caldwell's compact and wide-ranging musings are wry, surprising, and fresh."   —Amy Fusselman, author of *The Means*

"Chloé Caldwell's *Trying* is a sly memoir of self-discovery and loss. It is an ode to the countless ways that we try: to love, to forgive, to heal, to parent, to grieve, to rebuild a life. What a humane and vulnerable book."   —Isle McElroy, author of *People Collide*

"*Trying* meets the reader at the intersection of fertility, creativity, and desire—I read it in long bursts, finding it nearly impossible to put down. Chloé Caldwell's writing is often profound and frequently electric—I loved this book."

—Chelsea Hodson, author of *Tonight I'm Someone Else*

"*Trying* reads like poetry and feels like a conversation with your coolest friend. In breaking the 'rules' of memoir, Chloé Caldwell has created something much greater. An extraordinary book."

—Molly Roden Winter, author of *More: A Memoir of Open Marriage*

Trying

Also by Chloé Caldwell

Legs Get Led Astray
Women: A Novella
I'll Tell You in Person
The Red Zone: A Love Story

Trying

A Memoir

Chloé Caldwell

Graywolf Press

Excerpt from *Liars* by Sarah Manguso reproduced with permission from the author.

Published by Graywolf Press
212 Third Avenue North, Suite 485
Minneapolis, Minnesota 55401

www.graywolfpress.org

Published in the United States of America
Printed in Canada

ISBN 978-1-64445-347-6   (paperback)
ISBN 978-1-64445-348-3   (ebook)

2 4 6 8 9 7 5 3 1
First Graywolf Printing, 2025

Library of Congress Cataloging-in-Publication Data

Names: Caldwell, Chloe, author.
Title: Trying : a memoir / Chloé Caldwell.
Description: Minneapolis : Graywolf Press, 2025.
Identifiers: LCCN 2024060288 (print) | LCCN 2024060289 (ebook) |
    ISBN 9781644453476 (trade paperback) | ISBN 9781644453483 (epub)
Subjects: LCSH: Caldwell, Chloe. | Authors, American—Biography—
    21st century. | Infertility, Female. | LCGFT: Autobiographies.
Classification: LCC PS3603.A432 Z46 2025 (print) |
    LCC PS3603.A432 (ebook) | DDC 814/.6—dc23/eng/20250205
LC record available at https://lccn.loc.gov/2024060288
LC ebook record available at https://lccn.loc.gov/2024060289

Cover design: Kimberly Glyder

For my dad, who taught me "you get good at what you do"

and for my friend JD Urban

My first batch of bread was a failure, but I ate it all.
And that makes it a success.

—Eva Baltasar, *Mammoth*

Author's note: This is a work of nonfiction. Some names and identifying details have been changed. Dialogue has been recreated from memory and text messages. Much has been omitted for stylistic purposes. In Act 3, some chronology is intentionally blurred and nonlinear, which reflects my experience and memory of that specific time period.

Trying

ACT I

It was fun for a while
There was no way of knowing
—*Roxy Music, "More Than This"*

On a winter morning my friend's kid hears me telling my friend about all the sticks I pee on.

"You pee on sticks?!" They are ovulation and pregnancy test sticks, but she is imagining me in the woods. Like a dog.

This is new: I run from pregnant people. When I see a pregnant person, I duck. Turn around. A glimpse of a stroller makes my body rotate away.

I celebrate Shabbat in the Old City of Jerusalem, Israel, where I am traveling with a group of thirty people for six days. The company brings "creatives" on themed trips: there are trips for sports, tech, pride, and music. The trip I am invited on is called Reality Storytellers.

The tour guide brings us to the Western Wall after we write our prayers. We can write as many as we like, he says, which surprises me for some reason, though I'm not sure where I got the idea you could only pray once. I write two prayers down. Some of the creatives with me know what I am praying for, even tell me what to pray for.

The walk to the wall from the street is dizzying and claustrophobic. We all wear white.

My prayer falls out of the wall. I watch it happen. I'm not sure what to do about it.

Celebrities who have announced pregnancies and given birth during the time I've been trying:

Ilana Glazer

Rihanna

Stephanie Beatriz

Maya Erskine

Iliza Shlesinger

Anna Konkle

Chloë Sevigny

Alanis Morissette (This one really stung for some reason.)

Emily Ratajkowski (This one too.)

Mandy Moore

Cameron Diaz

Gigi Hadid

Julia Stiles

Anne Hathaway

Daryl Hannah (This was fake news but I believed it for a while.)

Greta Gerwig

Rihanna again

We offer affordable and innovative ways to create your family, the hold message for the fertility clinic says over and over with classical music playing in the background. What if I don't want an innovative way to create my family? It reminds me of when I described a restaurant to a friend as having creative pizza and she said she just wanted regular pizza.

I steal pads whenever I'm at the fertility clinic because I'm really trying to maximize the perks.

I'm somewhat kidding about "trying," though I'm not sure what word to use in its place.

In an interview with David Letterman in the early 2000s, Amy Sedaris plopped down on the chair and said that she and her imaginary boyfriend were "trying." She talked about her imaginary boyfriend every time she went on Letterman. "It's so gross when people say that," she said. "*Trying.*"

Noncelebrities: An acquaintance. Friend from high school. Friend of a friend I do yoga with. A distant relative. A person I rode the bus with in elementary school. A writer. Another writer. An editor I used to work with. Someone on Instagram. Someone I sit next to on Amtrak. Someone's daughter. Someone's mother. A podcaster I follow. A publicist I follow. An editor I follow. Someone who sits next to me on Amtrak.

A text from my childhood best friend, who has also been trying for years: *Saw on Insta today the girl I used to babysit is pregnant with twins. That'll knock you down a few pegs.*

But. I was always the friend who went to yoga. Who brought an apple to lunch. At jobs in New York City, while others ordered takeout, I ate my brought-from-home lunch of an apple, carrots, and soup. I ate the diet of a horse. How ridiculous this line of thinking is. As if my lunches in 2008 should get me pregnant now.

Shouldn't they?

"In case you're unfamiliar with this particular feeling," Haley Nahman writes in her newsletter, "imagine if someone said you'd be receiving a life-changing phone call some time in the next year, but as soon as tomorrow, and that you may notice signs in your body when the call is imminent, although not necessarily. And if you eat poorly or drink too much or work out the wrong way or not enough, it may alter the quality of the news. Now tell me you wouldn't lose your mind just a little bit."

She talks about a friend who'd said the brain of someone trying to get pregnant should be studied.

Consider this book to be that brain.

Walking to a bougie-ass store five blocks from my apartment to purchase a card for my friend's baby shower, I pass three pregnant people. I know which card I want. It's a card I hate, the one that reads, "Holy Shit! You're Pregnant!"

Though I'm deciding between that card and one that says, "Holy Shit! You Made a Baby!"

I go with "Holy Shit! You're Pregnant!"

What would a card for me say? Holy Shit! You've Been Trying for Three Years and You're Not Pregnant! Holy Shit! You *haven't* made a baby! Holy shit! You're thirty-six! Almost thirty-seven! Holy Shit! That sucks! Holyshitholyshitholyshitholyshit!

The card costs seven dollars. Seven dollars for a stupid expression I could have written on a piece of paper for free.

When my mom was pregnant, she'd go to Friendly's for vanilla milkshakes. She craved them. At her mother-in-law's house, she looked in the mirror and lifted her shirt, and the moment she saw her breasts enlarged and veiny she knew. I want to have the same experience. I have lifted my shirt multiple times to induce the same experience. I was supposed to tell her, "Remember when you were at Grandma's house and went into the bathroom and looked at your breasts and you knew you were pregnant? The same thing happened to me!" I was supposed to be able to say, "Mom, didn't you crave vanilla milkshakes from Friendly's when you were pregnant? I've been craving them!"

On the sidewalk outside the boutique where I work on weekends, there is a chalkboard sign that reads, LIFE CHANGING PANTS. All day, people, mostly tourists from New York City, Connecticut, Boston, and Philadelphia, sometimes from San Francisco and Seattle, come in to ask about the sign.

My friend works down the street, and we text each other what customers say about themselves. If you thought body positivity was alive and well, work one day in a shop that specializes in pants.

"The fit wasn't great for my weird body."

"I did a lot of grief eating over the winter."

"I wouldn't like how I looked in a picture."

"When I lose ten pounds I'll come back for them."

"These belts are the same size, right? Not for fatties like me but I'll lose the weight."

"I look too slutty."

"I haven't been a size small since 2008."

"Do I have camel toe?"

"Do I look too slutty?"

"Size XL is a scary term."

"They're probably not life-changing for small Asian women like me."

"I'm roly-poly so they'd never fit me."

"You have to be tall to wear these."

"You have to have a long torso to wear these."

"You have to have a short torso to wear these."

"I have no butt."

"I have no hips."

"I have no boobs."

"If I wear all white, I look like I'm getting ready to give someone a Pap smear."

"If I tried on the white ones, I'd look like a big fat ice cream truck."

"I have a huge butt like JLo."

"I have the weirdest torso."

This negative body talk really weighs on me, my friend texts.

I'm drained by it at the end of the day, I text back.

Just try them on, I tell everyone. One day I want to count the number of times I say "try" but it's too many.

I think about changing the sign from LIFE CHANGING PANTS to LIFE CHANGING PANTS (IF YOU KEEP AN OPEN MIND). It isn't my store, though, so I can't.

If the store didn't have cameras and the owner couldn't see me, I'd definitely bring the life-changing-pants sign inside each day, probably in the afternoon when the burnout begins. *You* try convincing someone a pair of pants will change their life all day.

People say stuff is "life-changing" all the time: brands of moisturizer, suitcases, shoes, candle warmers, headphones, tarot cards, at-home eyebrow tint. It reminds me of one of my students, who used to be addicted to crack and who told me she notices how often people say, "It's like crack," about everything. Dairy-free ice cream, popcorn, cereal, a certain type of cracker, granola, cheese, kombucha, chocolate. "Well, it's good . . . but it's not like *crack*," my student said. "Only crack is like crack."

The fertility clinic should swap slogans with the boutique. What if the boutique's sign was INNOVATIVE AND AFFORDABLE PANTS and the fertility clinic's hold recording and slogan was, "Life-changing ways to create your family"?

I stroll into a gift store, only to be assaulted with mom phrases. The necklaces read:

MAMA

WORLD'S OKAYEST MAMA

C-SECTION

MAMA BEAR

MAMA-TO-BE

My favorite is the martyrish tote bag: NOTHING IN THIS BAG BELONGS TO ME. Mom Life.

Then put something of yours in the goddamn bag. Throw a ChapStick in there, a water bottle, a pen. There you go, now something in there belongs to you.

An acupuncturist refuses to work on me postovulation because if it's in there "you want it to stick." Another acupuncturist tells me the previous acupuncturist is wrong. An acupuncturist tells me to stop drinking coffee. Coffee tightens you when you should be flowing. An acupuncturist tells me if I'm really a "stress ball" but not telling him, then I won't get pregnant. Another one says to keep your midriff and ankles always covered. All the acupuncturists tell me my pulses are great and getting pregnant won't be a problem. The acupuncturists say to eat warm food, to keep water on the counter and not in the fridge. To eat wet breakfasts. I already knew this, though. My whole life my mom has said the phrase "room temp." One acupuncturist lives up the road from where I grew up. I see it as a sign that she is the person who will get me pregnant, but then she goes to Nepal and decides to stay forever. Another acupuncturist tells me to stay warm and drink bone broth. Another tells me to always keep my ankles and midriff covered. My mom pays for my acupuncture; it's a pity pay, I think, though I still appreciate it. We both thought this would have ended by now.

The acupuncturist who moved to Nepal tells me that since I write books I know how to bring things to fruition. That is fertility, she says. She tells me to make a shrine with a candle and things from the natural world. I have some driftwood and add some stones I'd collected. She also says to deliver the shrine warm milk every morning.

"Nah that's too weird," a friend says when I tell her about the milk, and we laugh.

The new acupuncturist I jibe with. She's a twenty-five-minute drive into the woods and specializes in the menstrual cycle and fertility. I see her for a year and a half and then she discloses to me that she is pregnant. "It's hard to tell my clients this," she says.

"I'm happy for you," I say, because I am, and because it is the thing to say, and because I know, intellectually, that one person's pregnancy doesn't take away the chances of another person getting pregnant. This is what happens in life! People get pregnant!

Nonetheless, I fall apart when I get home. She is twenty-four weeks along when she tells me. It feels like the scene in *Mrs. Doubtfire* when Sally Field's character finds out Robin Williams has been masking as Mrs. Doubtfire.

"The whole time?"

"The whole time?"

"The whole time?"

I didn't notice because whenever I walk in she is sitting at a desk, and then I immediately lie down on the acupuncture bed and see only her face.

Still, before she told me, part of me knew. She is of a certain age. I want to say of course she is pregnant; she's an acupuncturist. But my childhood best friend, the one also experiencing the trying of it all, tells me her acupuncturist has had multiple failed IUIs and, like me, doesn't want to do IVF.

She seems pretty defeated, she writes.

A few years ago, I was in Sayulita, Mexico, for a friend's fortieth birthday. She wanted to go paddle boarding in the ocean. I am not athletic at all, but I decided to challenge myself. Friends kept telling me I'd be good at it since I have good balance from yoga. I made it to the ocean with my paddleboard, then panicked the minute we began trying to get on our boards. There were sharp rocks and waves. I wouldn't even try. I gave up before anyone else did. A similar thing happened the first time I tried kayaking. (Why, for both of these activities, was my first time in the ocean, not on a lake? Or a pond? Water that is still instead of unpredictable?)

My friend paddle boarded every day and ended up with sea lice all over her hands and feet from the moldy board.

So.

In the trying-to-conceive forums online, people call the vaginal ultrasound wand "the dildo cam." One day I google "dildo cam" in hopes of reading funny stories. It doesn't occur to me that searching "dildo cam" will bring up loads of pornography, and that now my phone will serve me related ads.

Later, the dildo cam will become an anecdote I can tell not-super-close friends over cheese and wine, when we are speaking of Pap smears and women's health and doctors. They won't know the reason I've had it so often. I will be able to hold court and the friends will burst into laughter together, having no idea of everything that's underneath. Anecdotally, it's funny. In my reality, it's a tragedy.

Sometimes I forget that the Reddit trying-to-conceive community isn't called TTC since so many other forums are. I remember, though, as soon as I type it in and it brings me to the Toronto Transit Commission.

"I'm curious what pants will change my life," one customer says cynically when she walks through the door.

"At least you're curious!" I say.

"Which are the life-changing pants?" another asks.

"All of them!" I say. I should say: "It depends how you want your life to change."

Overheard as two women enter the store, one walking with a cane and in her eighties:

"I hate my cane. It's so ugly."

Her daughter: "Okay, Mom, we'll get you a sexier cane."

Here's the thing: the pants actually *are* life-changing. I mean, they haven't gotten me pregnant, but still.

One woman walks in the store and drops a few thousand dollars. When I ask if she'd like a receipt, she says, "No. I want to pretend this never happened."

In the beginning, friends would text: *You haven't been on social media so I thought maybe you were pregnant.* Early on, another friend in the dressing room with me said, "You gotta get a baby in there," pointing to my stomach.

"I'm working on it," I responded.

But after a certain number of months into years, they stopped asking. Now they say, "How's that going?" apprehensively. Avoid your eyes when someone else announces their pregnancy at your birthday party. Things become silent the way a city does in a snowstorm.

No one calls cancer unexplained. Or a divorce unexplained. Or a broken leg unexplained. What about calling a novel that doesn't get finished or published unexplained? And if something is *unexplained*, isn't it a writer's job to attempt to explain it? To at least try?

My friend is a nephrologist at Columbia, and I text him my thoughts on the diagnosis of unexplained infertility—how the term "unexplained" isn't used for anything else. He writes: *We usually say "idiopathic" to denote unexplained but idiopathic makes us sound smarter and keep a distance of expertise between us and patients, but for some reason there's never been a reason to use idiopathic with infertility, we use unexplained.*

In 2012, I was in the passenger seat while a guy I was dating drove. His sister sat in the back seat. They'd asked me what I'd done that day, and I described meeting someone for coffee who'd wanted to meet me for coffee because she'd read one of my books.

"That's so cool," the sister said. "I wonder why people never invite me to get coffee."

"Be more interesting," the guy I was dating said, and cracked up.

His sister was offended. I thought it was funny.

But I am not *interesting* anymore. I go to dinner with one of my favorite comedians and I only talk about *trying*. We could have been talking about books! Film! Relationships! Whatever else people talk about! But I drone on about not getting pregnant. Characters in nineties movies are addicted to saying about men that they're only interested in one thing, but what about a person who wants a baby and can think of nothing else?

Supposedly the definition of insanity is to do the same thing over and over but expect different results, but isn't that precisely what trying to get pregnant and failing is?

Is it actually failing, though? And if so, isn't everyone always saying to fail better? I hate that phrase. Cycles of not getting pregnant are called "failed cycles." When do they go from being cycles to being failed?

Mimetic theory says that we mimic others' desires. But I'm not mimicking anyone's desire to have a child. I want to have a child because I want to have a child.

I'm sitting on the couch with a friend. She says, "Maybe your sperm and egg aren't . . . compatible?"

She isn't a doctor and this isn't an actual thing. But I get what she means.

Somewhere, I read the quote, "Some delays are protection."

Bill Burr has a bit where he makes fun of Oprah for introducing a guest as being a mother, which she says we all know "is the most difficult job on the planet." "Any job that you can do in your pajamas is not a difficult job," Burr says.

I'm supposed to take offense to this joke, but I tend to agree. It applies to both mothering and writing.

It's weird when I go on Instagram and see someone who had a baby watching my Insta story regularly. I think that if I had had a baby I would be freed from such peasant activities. I know that's bullshit, and of course habits like scrolling don't go away and of course you scroll when you can't sleep or the baby is sleeping or breastfeeding. Still, I judge these new mothers. They judge me too.

On a Sunday afternoon, I sit on a small beach, reading. A woman's son, maybe one and a half years old, with blue eyes, walks toward me. He does this about three times, just walks over and smiles or looks up at the sky and points. He isn't bothering anyone, yet his mom is embarrassed. Whenever he begins to even look in my direction she tries to get him to stay near her. I think if he were my son, I'd let him walk up to people without being embarrassed and hovering, but I know I'm probably wrong.

It reminds me of "By Song, Not Album," an essay Hannah Tennant-Moore published in 2009:

> One day on the bus I sat in front of a little girl wearing a pink raincoat. We were riding by the Seine, and the girl asked her mother, "Est-ce qu'il y a des dauphins là, Maman?"

"Non, il n'y a pas de dauphins."

I thought that if she'd been my daughter, I would have answered, "Yes, perhaps there are some dolphins in the Seine."

In the movie *White Oleander*, fifteen-year-old Astrid's biological mother goes to prison for a murder. When she meets the foster parent played by Renée Zellweger, we see her smiling for the first time. There is a scene where Renée Zellweger meets Michelle Pfeiffer, the biological mother. Cruelly, Michelle Pfeiffer says to Renée Zellweger, about Astrid: "She must be such a comfort to you, not being able to have children of your own." That night, sleeping in the same bed as Astrid, Renée Zellweger's character kills herself, overdosing on pills. Because she couldn't have a biological child? Was she depressed because of that or was she already depressed and this exacerbated her depression? What are we supposed to think?

In the movie *Raising Arizona*, when Holly Hunter and Nicolas Cage return the baby they kidnapped, Holly Hunter says, "I just wanted to be a mama." The father of the baby she has stolen says something actually helpful: "If you can't have kids, you just keep trying, and hope medical science catches up with you."

I always thought Charlotte was the most tragic *Sex and the City* character. It was unjust that she wasn't able to get pregnant when the others were child-free by choice.

The plotline for Stephanie in *Fuller House* is that she can't get pregnant, so she uses Kimmy Gibbler as a surrogate. Kimmy Gibbler as surrogate! I always knew she had a good heart.

Watching *And Just Like That . . .*, the *Sex and the City* reboot, I am baffled to see Charlotte did in fact have a biological child in addition to her adopted daughter. I have to search the web to learn she'd ended up conceiving naturally in one of the *Sex and the City* movies.

This detail hadn't stuck with me, hadn't moved me then, because until you are actively trying and failing to become pregnant, you don't care. Back then, for me, Charlotte could have been saying she ate eggs for breakfast.

In the film *Private Life*, Kathryn Hahn plays a married forty-year-old writer opting to do in vitro fertilization. When her husband suggests that she prioritized different aspects of her life over getting pregnant, she yells, "A lot of women get pregnant at forty. I thought I could too!" I was thirty-two when I watched the movie.

In the British show *Trying*, a couple explores various paths like fostering and adopting, because IVF won't work for them for a reason they don't disclose on the show. In one scene, the character Nikki asks her mom, "What's it like to have kids? To have all this?" She gestures to her sister trying on wedding dresses.

"It's like the sun on your back," her mom responds.

On *Friends*, Monica is diagnosed with a term not used anymore: the "inhospitable environment" of her womb. Chandler is also said to have low-motility/lazy sperm, but the blame is mostly placed on Monica's hostile womb.

I come up with an actionable plan for them. Don't they know Chandler could take CoQ10 and ashwagandha and fish oil and clean up his eating habits? Don't they know about exercise? Don't they know that sperm regenerates every sixty days? Don't they know to get tested more than once? Don't they know about Athletic Greens, for god's sake? My husband B's sperm count was low at first but after these changes it went up.

But they didn't have Google. Discord. Reddit. It was the nineties. A diagnosis was an end instead of a beginning.

I mean, I know *Friends* needed the plot point, but they aren't even going to *try*? They just accept it and have a superquick conversation about how they're going to adopt.

In another episode, Phoebe gets a positive pregnancy test the same day as an embryo transfer. This is impossible. If you do test positive, it would be because of the medication and would be a false positive.

I shouldn't expect the writers of *Friends* to know all of this. I just wish I didn't have to know it all, either.

Most of the people who come in the shop assume I want them to buy something. I have "store-owner energy." It can be awkward when they ask, "Is this your store?" and I just say, "Nope," because I'm not sure what else to say. So I add, "I'm just a fan."

"Enjoy your pants," I sometimes say when people are leaving the store with a purchase, and then immediately feel like a moron.

Sometimes, if the customer really did want to buy something but the pants didn't work out and they feel bad, I say, "You gave it a really good shot."

Whenever a woman writes a book with her personal story, she has to bring in an alternate element of nature and then her book will be more popular, because the readers feel smart. Hawks, stars, water/ swimming, Greek mythology. If not, she has to bring in academic jargon.

What could my element of nature be, so that people will take my book seriously? So that they will feel it is worth reading? Cranes? Trees? Koalas? Whales? Weather? There are so many options. Why can't I just choose one? My thoughts are not enough, I agree.

People say to write what you know, but when you do write what you know, you're treated like a psycho.

My alternative element, I suppose, is working retail, but retail doesn't seem *literary* enough.

When I teach writing, I tell my students about the revision trick where you scan through whatever you've written to make sure each paragraph begins differently. I do the same thing at the boutique— different variations of "hi" and "bye" and "have a nice day" and "enjoy your Sunday" and "have a good evening" and "take care." One day I describe a jumpsuit as "bra-friendly" and a woman bursts out laughing. She says she has never heard that before. I say that actually all our overalls and jumpsuits and tops are bra-friendly. I picture a jumpsuit being friendly to bras, greeting them and being warm.

I scroll Instagram and see a pregnancy announcement. Two gay women—one I'd met at a residency over five years ago. It's been years since I've liked or commented on pregnancy posts. I don't leave shining stars and heart eyes. It feels fake, so I just pretend I don't see the posts. This is one way I have changed from my former self. I googled both their ages. Googling ages is my hobby, my salve, my passion.

Joan Didion and Emily Bernard and Jillian Lauren adopted. Michelle Obama did IVF. What was wrong with Obama's sperm? It became popular in 2020 and 2021 to ask what lived "rent-free" in your head. Now you know what lives in mine.

How do you know when you're done? A question I hear weekly in my writing classes. Usually I respond that it's an instinct.

Though I agree that writing a book is mysterious, there is much more you can control than trying to conceive. If you wake up every day and write a thousand words, you will eventually have fifty thousand words. You will have a book, even if it's a bad book.

If you wake up every day and have sex with someone who has sperm, you may or may not be pregnant at the end of it. You may not have a baby. Even a bad one.

A close friend tells me, "Your books *mother* so many people!" As if I give a shit.

One of my friends understands, because she's had experience with both books and babies. "A book is a small consolation when it's a baby you want," she says.

There's a piece of writing online called "Your Book Might Not Sell, and You Have to Live With That." I share it occasionally with students, but feel sort of mean when I do, since I have published books. It feels like a person with children sharing an article with me called "You Might Not Get Pregnant, and You Have to Live With That."

I see that someone is teaching a class on conceiving a book. I conceived this book because I'm not conceiving. I could also teach a class on conceiving.

How to Conceive a Book When You Can't Conceive
Carving Out Space in the Infertility Literary World
What to Expect When You're Not Expecting
What to Expect When You Don't Know What to Expect
What to Expect When You Were Expecting to Get Pregnant
Fertility Accountability
Conceiving Better

In her song "My Baby Wants a Baby," Annie Clark (stage name St. Vincent) sings, "But I wanna play guitar all day / Make all my meals in microwaves." She says she won't have any legacy if she has a baby. (She doesn't, in the song or in real life.) "Then I couldn't stay in bed all day," she says, meaning if she had a baby.

Yeah, you couldn't stay in bed all day, I think, but you would also have a baby.

It's like those scenes of Greta Gerwig and Adam Driver in the film *Frances Ha*. Adam Driver's character tries showing Greta Gerwig's character a video of someone on a motorcycle and she shakes her head. "Motorcycles are so loud."

"What?"

"I mean, you can't listen to music when you're on a motorcycle."

"But you're on a *motorcycle*," Adam Driver's character responds.

And later: "We could go to a movie."

"Movies are so expensive now."

"Yeah . . . but you're at the *movies*."

A woman I meet tells me she refers to her daughter as her "vagina ripper." It is so much easier to speak to strangers about wanting a child. I tell her about forty being my cutoff. I say I won't have the energy after that. I've given this spiel to lots of people, friends, therapists, but this woman is the first person to challenge it. She explains, "If that's God's plan, then you will find the energy. Don't cut yourself off."

I've been telling my students the same thing. They all want to write fifteen-hundred-word pieces because they think anything longer can't be published. "Don't cut yourself off!" I say. When did everyone forget that long-form essays and books are a thing? If you're cutting yourself off, you're not even getting to what might be the good stuff. You're stopping too soon. You need to write a shit ton, and then cut. They tell me their pieces are bloated or long-winded. What I don't understand is how people expect to write books if they keep stopping themselves from writing.

It's not that I don't understand constraint. Constraint gives me a sense of control in a world of chaos the way makeovers give Cher in *Clueless* a sense of control in a world of chaos. Constraint is good. This book is full of constraint and omission. But constraining length is different. Don't you ever wonder what would happen if you kept going? What sentences you might write? What revelations you might have? What books could come out of you?

No matter what I say about the life-changing pants, I get a laugh. I suppose people aren't even listening to what I say. They're just ready to laugh. A good audience, I suppose. "You guys have been a great audience!" I should yell when they leave, the way comedians do at the ends of their live sets.

I've recently worked on my pitch to make sure I mention that it's a woman-owned and woman-run company and that everything is made in New York City.

"Where in New York City?" they challenge me.

"The Garment District."

"I didn't think clothes were still made there."

Most people probably don't need to take a Klonopin before going to a friend's baby shower. I am not most people anymore. Five of us are around the table for brunch, and everyone else has children. I am the one-in-five statistic of infertility at the table. I have my period and when we finish brunch I go home and make mac and cheese and bleed more.

A note I jot down: *random, cruel, and out of my control.* I had heard it somewhere.

Walking down the street, my friend and I see a license plate: PREGNANT. My friend takes a photo of it; he can't believe how insane this license plate is, but I'm used to living in this world.

Six months later, a different friend who lives in the town posts a photo of the same car and license plate. They caption it "Bro."

In yoga, my teacher says she is celebrating failure.

When I first started peeing on the ovulation sticks, it was just for fun. A novelty. A joke. Like when my dad cooked French toast years ago and my brother said, "Since when do we have whipped cream on French toast?" And my dad responded, "It was a joke." My friend had given me some extras she had after getting pregnant. I didn't know how to use them and would do them at night or at random times of the day, when I wasn't even ovulating. The process became more refined over the years. I learned to do them only in the morning, starting around day seven of my cycle. I always got positives. Sometimes I bought the digital ones that gave you a circle when you weren't ovulating, a blinking smiley face when you were getting close, and a solid smiley face on the day you were. They took five minutes to load, so often they'd be lying around my apartment, a stick with a smiley face.

Where the sticks have traveled with me: Lincoln, Massachusetts. Denver, Colorado. Vail, Colorado. Aspen, Colorado. Messejana, Portugal. Lisbon, Portugal. Sayulita, Mexico. Yelapa, Mexico. And why? All they've done is generate trash.

We all know the narrative: Person gets pregnant when they stop trying. People absolutely love this story, but what's funny is you can't actually get pregnant without trying.

In "Preparing for a Baby on the Brink of Apocalypse," Chelsea Martin writes, "I was still determined to have an accidental pregnancy, like my mother and her mother and all the mothers that came before us."

In her memoir *In the Dream House*, Carmen Maria Machado writes, "Every television show you watched in your twenties included some kind of mystical pregnancy. Every interesting female character needs one, or so the showrunners seem to think." I know what she means by a mystical pregnancy: unexpected, unplanned, a good surprise, or against all odds. TV raised me to think I'd have a mystical pregnancy too. I'd get pregnant at the most perfectly imperfect time. I was positive that was how people's lives went.

On the website *Romper*, under Menu, there is a section called Pregnancy. Underneath are the subcategories: Trying, Birth, and After. I click the Trying drop-down, looking for essays and people's stories and camaraderie, but the only essay I see is my own.

Ambivalence, ambivalence, ambivalence. All the mothers and maybe-wannabe mothers write about ambivalence. It's the motherhood buzzword. It is popular to admit that you agonized over the choice and came around to wanting a child. But I have never had ambivalence about having a child. Can the inverse happen? Wanting, wanting, wanting, and coming around to ambivalence?

There seem to be three popular categories: momfluencers, the ambivalent, and IVF doers. Where's my group?

The cool girls don't want to give up their writing time. I'd happily give up some writing time. I've been writing for fifteen years and am ready to give some of it up.

There's a joke Chelsea Peretti tells about not having children: "What are we supposed to do otherwise? Keep going out to dinner?"

I have coffee with a friend who has given up coffee, because everyone seems to be giving up coffee. She is a musician, forty-three. She is still deciding whether she should try to have kids for one more year. She's been making music since her early twenties. We agree we are sick of doing our art. That we did life in reverse, art first and babies later, unlike a lot of people we talk to who have kids but feel creatively stunted.

Another friend has a debut upmarket murder novel she wants to sell; she's taking it out to agents soon. She's forty-one. "If I can't get an agent or get my book published, that's the only way I'll decide to have a baby." We crack up. A year later she ends up selling her novel and, true to her word, she becomes less interested in having kids and more interested in her author photo. She orders twelve navy blue sweaters to make sure she has the perfect one for her photo, and we laugh our asses off.

Before I was trying, maybe eight years ago, I met a newly separated friend for a drink. I'd known him and his wife for years, and he disclosed that they weren't able to get pregnant. On our barstools I asked him if that was part of why they separated. He paused, thought for a while. Then he said, "I think it made us see sides of each other we wouldn't have otherwise seen."

Until it happens to *you*, you don't care about different hardships, my mom explains at a family dinner. Cancer, Covid, Alzheimer's, auto-immune disorders, infertility, dementia. "Until it happens to *you*," she emphasizes. "Until it happens to you or someone you love," she adds.

It isn't the babies who scare me when I avoid strollers. It's the people pushing them. There's this smugness to them, the same smugness I want to have.

One morning a friend texts me: *You are so lucky you're not a parent.* She knows I want kids, and I love that she texts me this. The same day she texts, *I want you to have a kid,* and her juxtaposition of those two texts delights me.

I finally decide to go to the foster parent website.

Do you have extra space in your heart and home?

Actually, no. We don't have an extra bedroom.

Well, that was delightfully efficient! I close the browser.

ACT II

Hope is a dangerous thing for a woman like me to have
but I have it

—*Lana Del Rey, "hope is a dangerous thing for
a woman like me to have—but i have it"*

The morning of my first intrauterine insemination, the answer to Wordle is "mourn." I don't play Wordle. My husband B does, though.

On my phone, where I kept a list of baby names, there is now a list of what I can do if the IUI doesn't work:

Iced coffee
Wine, tattoo?
Teeth whitening, manicure, blowout
Watch the new Amy Schumer show and get Thai or Mexican takeout

I never get manicures or blowouts because of the chemicals and coffee and wine are the devil, according to the acupuncturists. I drink water and lemon in the morning, sometimes a green tea. If I eat and drink perfectly, minimally, I'll get rewarded, is how my brain thinks.

For years these were the images of getting pregnant that ran through my head: Running out onto the street squealing in ecstasy. Calling my mom from the bathroom. A trying-too-hard social media photo where my hair was long and bump was big. Or maybe an effortless photo. Regardless, there'd be a photo.

Now there are images I hadn't known even existed, and they are becoming memories, like handing my credit card across the counter to pay for an IUI.

IUI, I had decided, was noninvasive enough for me. It only takes a couple of minutes. Plus, my insurance covers the blood work and monitoring. With my insurance, the procedure itself is $250 (it can range anywhere from $250 to $4,000) and my mom treats me on her L.L.Bean credit card. Because even if one is experiencing what our culture calls infertility, one should always use the opportunity to get their Bean Bucks.

"What is for others nature / is for us culture," Edward Hirsch writes in his poem "The Welcoming."

It's basically the turkey-baster method, but medical. The person trying to get pregnant is given medication such as Clomid, which helps the body ovulate more than the normal one egg per month. After four days, the person goes to the clinic for the dildo cam, which shows how many follicles (follicles turn into eggs) there are.

The first time I got checked after Clomid, the nurse seemed proud of me. I had four mature follicles. "You took to the medicine so well," she said, as if I'd done something more impressive than swallow pills.

After they've checked for your multiple follicles, the clinic has you order the trigger shot from a pharmacy. It ships to you in a box containing a needle filled with the chemical HCG. You give yourself the trigger shot, which will make you ovulate. B doesn't help, saying he's scared of needles, so you do it in the bedroom while he makes dinner.

The actual inserting of the sperm happens early in the morning after the trigger shot. It takes about the same time as a Pap smear. You have to go to the clinic two hours early to drop the sperm off for sperm washing.

When the nurse is putting the sperm in, she calls it "the sample." "Here comes the sample," she says. Kind of like when you are feeding a baby and you say, "Here comes the airplane!"

Most people go cuckoo waiting for results after that, but these days it's my favorite part. It's the only time I can solidly live in uncertainty, unknowing. The only time I can relax, because I've done all I can do. My friends and everyone in my Discord group are so impressed with how I don't start testing eight days past ovulation, but I wish I could live in limbo for longer. The two-week wait is cozy. Maybe pregnant, maybe not. Probably, probably not. Je ne sais pas. It's the only time I'm released from planning anything—a period, an ovulation, a drive to the clinic. It's up to the body now.

Sixteen days after the IUI, you're supposed to go back to the clinic for blood work. After the blood work, always done between 7:00 a.m. and 9:00 a.m., you drive home. Or if you're me, you drive to Trader Joe's for instant miso ramen and half-and-half with the cute drawing of a cow on it and frozen taquitos and then you drive home. You feel superproductive because you've already driven an hour, had blood drawn, and grocery shopped, and it's not even nine. A few hours later you'll get a phone call telling you whether you're pregnant—if there is HCG in your blood. You walk around subtly elated all day, having a secret from everyone.

The call comes after 3:00 p.m. I can tell by the tone of the nurse's voice. Reined in, neutral. Slightly apologetic. The IUI didn't work. She sounds exasperated, small. She probably has to give news like this all day.

"On paper everything is perfect," she adds, "so we don't know what is going on."

Of course I like this anecdote; it redeems me. For the next couple of years I can say, *Even the doctors are stumped.* Or repeat, *On paper everything is perfect.*

Once the pandemic started, we'd rearranged a tiny back room that we used as storage into an office for me. It is packed to the brim with crap: tchotchkes, snow pants and boots, an enormous filing cabinet, books, folding chairs, art that needs to be hung.

The roof back there starts leaking whenever there is a heavy rain or snowstorm. It starts over the holidays, and B doesn't want to bother our landlord, who would have to call the roof guy. So I just live like this, moving my books and journals and papers around so they won't get ruined. But hearing the consistent drips and drops makes me extremely irritated.

When I learn that ingredients like "fragrance" might be the reason I'm not getting pregnant, I spend days and days with every cosmetic product in my home laid on the living room rug. I find a company that accepts donations for incarcerated women. I package them all up and send them out of my house, positive that I have figured out the issue. Of course now I'll get pregnant. I download apps that let me point my phone camera at products and rate them from not harmful to most harmful. Shopping and choosing shampoo and conditioner and bubble bath takes forever now, because almost everything is harmful.

I start to notice that when I see two cishet people walking together, they look wrong to me. Men and women look weird. Women and women or women and nonbinary people look right.

When I mention it to B, he says it is "interesting."

It's hard to wrap my mind around the fact I'm having a doctor medically insert sperm into me instead of having sex with B. In an essay I publish on the topic, I write that most people who post in the Reddit group r/TryingForABaby (138K members) are straight couples. One day when I asked about IUI, someone directed me to r/queerception (14K members), saying there was an abundance of knowledge around IUI in that space. I wouldn't say the r/TryingForABaby people kicked me out, exactly, but it did feel meaningful that they told me I wasn't in the right place.

So I left the hetero r/TryingForABaby group, where everyone talked about doing the BD (baby dance) with their DH (dear husband). Where most of the women were doing IVF and dismissed IUI because it has only 20 percent success rates.

I purchase a book called *The Queerness of Memory* because the title is perfect and the shade of green is soothing.

A woman comes in the shop to ask about the life-changing pants. Her response to the sign is: "That. Is. Sooooooooooo. Fuuuuuuuuuuuny," which she repeats over and over as she walks around. She says it slowly. She doesn't want to try pants on. She just wants to say how funny the sign is.

On slow days, or during the winter season, I do a lot of catching up on texts from friends. I won't even be thinking about infertility while texting, but then I go to write the word "imagine," or "interesting," and it autocorrects to "infertility" or "IVF."

"Why are the pants life-changing?"

"They're ninety-eight percent cotton and two percent stretch. Made in New York City. Flattering for all bodies, runs from XXS to 4XL. We're the only store in town that is size inclusive."

"Why are the pants life-changing?"

"You really have to try them on to understand."

"You got me in because of the sign."

"Yeah, we have some pretty great pants. Want to try a pair?"

"Life-changing pants, huh?"

"Yes! They're amazing. I'm wearing them now. They're so flattering and comfortable and made in New York. Ninety-eight percent cotton and two percent spandex. Let me know if you have any questions or want to try on a pair. You can see what they look like on me." I stand up to model.

"I was just kidding," they say.

"Oh. Sorry."

I attend a writers residency for two weeks in southern Portugal, in a farming town called Messejana, a word that means "prison." B is supposed to fly in for the second week, but he says his passport got stolen on the plane. I befriend another writer, an Armenian poet from Los Angeles. One night after splitting a bottle of wine, she wants to get cigarettes, because we are in Europe and they're cheap, though they may hurt her fertility, she says. She and her partner have been considering children. I laugh and tell her not to live her life based on her hypothetical fertility. But also, I'm a hypocrite and every day I live my life based on my hypothetical fertility.

After the residency I fly to Lisbon. Alone, I eat dinner at a café called Bistrô Gato Pardo. Bread, cheese, meatballs, a pureed vegetable soup. I count the kids as they walk by. Four toddlers. One small girl in a gray beret. A ten-or-so-year-old with a yo-yo. I take a photo of graffiti that says, "queer" in lowercase. The "q" is made into an eye. I post it on Instagram stories.

I write in my journal: *My self-worth is tied up completely in my fertility. I can barely enjoy a margarita without thinking about it.* Later I write: *I pray I'm getting closer to getting pregnant. Maybe I should start praying!*

In an essay, "The Anxiety of Being the Non-Bio Parent," Samantha Mann coins a term: "belly envy." She explains that it's a "lesbian-specific Freudian self-diagnosis," being envious of the partner who is carrying. But I was envious of everyone who was carrying, especially strangers.

In her memoir *Black Is the Body*, Emily Bernard writes about accepting and embracing her decision to adopt two daughters: "Still, when I stand next to pregnant women, my stomach sometimes feels concave and hollow."

A few friends and past students are announcing their divorces on Instagram. I am intrigued by one in particular, which begins: "Nora Ephron said never marry a man you wouldn't want to be divorced from." She goes on to explain that she and her husband are moving on to phase two of their relationship. She writes, "In short—I'm gay."

I show it to B and my mom. "This is how people announce their divorces now!" I say to my mom, divorced herself.

The cadence of her funny perfect blunt sentence sticks with me like an echo and makes me laugh. "In short—I'm gay." Often it pops into my head unexpectedly.

Even if a book ends without a baby, a quick google will often show you that the author has had a baby via IVF. Will I be one of these authors?

It is a dark feeling to look up writers and celebrities and feel disappointed that they now have children, because I should feel hopeful and happy for them, and I do. But I also feel betrayed.

If you search for "[insert writer's name] children," one of the results will be a Wikipedia page and underneath where the first couple of lines are excerpted it will say, Missing: ~~children~~ Show results with: children.

The longing itself is addictive, too. The longing is a *place*. If the longing goes away, what will I be left with?

The fertility clinic I go to is nothing like the ones in the films. In the movies they're usually crowded, with white walls and male doctors. In real life, there is carpet and not a soul in the waiting room. For the year and a half I went there I only met women. Women at the reception desk, women who took my blood, women who used the lubed-up dildo cam on me, women who inserted sperm.

When you take Clomid you have to sign a form agreeing that you're aware there is a risk of having twins. It can also induce psychosis; there's academic articles about it, people writing about it on the internet. But when I tell the doctors I went insane on Clomid—that I smashed a ceramic mug, couldn't leave bed—they just say I must be sensitive. In my Notes app:

Clomid diaries
Day 3
A blood moon last night
Storm today
Full moon tonight
I'm in the thick of it
Help

Have you ever looked in the mirror during an acid or psilocybin trip and your face looked like a Picasso painting? I begin to think that I have no control of my life; my voice changes; my hand doesn't look like it's my hand. I walk from room to room, moaning, sobbing, hyperventilating. I can actually feel my ovaries twinging, growing. If they say giving birth is the most natural thing in the world, Clomid is the opposite. On Clomid I yell things like, "Let's just get divorced!"

I've heard that pineapple is the universal (in)fertility symbol. But I don't subscribe. If I do I will see signs everywhere, become hopeful, become disappointed. Become hopeful, become disappointed. Become hopeful, become disappointed. I don't want to walk by stupid pineapple-patterned clothing at Target and think about infertility. Infertility doesn't need to ruin pineapple, a fruit I like. On Reddit, someone says she tried so hard to get pregnant that she ate a fuck ton of bromelain supplements for the fertility perks and she made herself ill.

If handling disappointment is a sign of emotional maturity (Is it? It should be.) then I am *off the charts.*

Turns out the pineapple is specifically for the IVF community, not even for general infertility. What is the symbol for trying for four years but bowing out of IVF? What is the symbol for unexplained infertility?

Customers can say all they want about the life-changing-pants sign, but the joke is on them when they end up wearing the pants straight out of the store, their other non-life-changing pants crumpled up and rejected in one of our bags. I get scissors and cut the tag out, the way I do for my stepdaughter. It feels intimate and tender, and I go the extra step to make sure the plastic tag holder is gone too, so it doesn't scratch their lower back.

The leak has gotten worse. B is on tour, so I send him a photo and video of the eight bowls and pots I have on the floor and on shelves. There is a strip of wood on the ceiling that has consistent drips along its entire length. Each morning I dump the full bowls in the sink and all day I walk and step over the bowls as though they were pets, sleeping cats.

Two friends and I are out for pizza and beer. One of the friends has fallen pregnant, unplanned. The other has a three-year-old. I know this sounds like a riddle, but it isn't.

The friend with the unplanned pregnancy already has a son, a nine-year-old. She isn't having an abortion and is conflicted though happy about being pregnant.

She looks at me and says, "I think you and I are both just having really bad luck." Her dark humor cheers me up.

I'm sitting in an overpriced mediocre café with my friend Layla, and she asks me what my plan is. Layla has been a way to mark the time. We met in a writing class in 2019. In 2020, she came to Hudson and we had drinks. Afterward, we took a walk and she told me she didn't want children, that she and her husband were happy with dogs. In 2021, she came to visit for a night. She'd changed her mind over the pandemic and had decided to go the medical route, because of her age and because she could afford it. In 2022, she did IVF and now she has a daughter.

"Just keep trying for the next few years, I guess. Keep doing what I'm doing."

She sort of laughs. She wants me to have more of a plan.

When I start doing IUIs, she seems relieved. It makes people uncomfortable that I'm not doing the obvious, the obvious being IVF.

The word "intervention" is used when we talk about this stuff. Medical intervention. Being intervened on.

When I pose the question to a group on Discord, of when they decided to pursue IVF, they say things like, "We didn't really have a choice." But of course you have a choice.

Write from an altered state: I've given this writing exercise dozens of times. A teacher gave it to my class, telling us that when she'd had her baby she was so tired and delirious she thought she'd never write again. She pushed herself to write from the tiredness, and found her writing became less precious that way, that she accessed a new place.

When I assign the exercise, I give the examples of having a migraine, having menstrual cramps, or writing at midnight when you normally write at 8:00 a.m. All those altered states are temporary. It only now occurs to me that this entire book is written from an altered state. An altered state that is prolonged—but also temporary.

Old Navy carries some legit knockoff life-changing pants. Their material is even the same: 98 percent cotton and 2 percent spandex. I am there for some inexpensive yoga clothes. I grab a couple pairs of pants and a tank top. As the cashier rings up the clothing, I watch each item pop up on the credit card reader. I notice one of the items is maternity pants. I had thought they were dance pants with a drop crotch. I tell the cashier I've changed my mind and don't need them.

At work, two customers come in and one tries on pants and one doesn't. The one who doesn't explains she is pregnant, which is why she can't. I stay cool, neutral. I have this conversation at least once a month with customers. A book I bought in my twenties at the Strand comes to mind: *Surviving Dreaded Conversations.*

I tell her that the demographic for the life-changing pants is the same as people who are pregnant or postpartum. This is true. The median age of the pants' popularity is thirty to forty-five. Many people who come in say they're the only pants they can wear postpregnancy because they're so comfortable.

"Yeah," the customer said. "I didn't even ask if you had maternity pants because it's so niche."

Is being pregnant . . . niche?

I have dinner with three childless friends. Two of them have frozen their eggs, a somewhat easy decision for them because their respective jobs at Etsy and CNN offer fertility coverage. I'm jealous, because if that was offered to me I'd do it too. I'm nothing if not an opportunist. I always tell my students to use their resources.

A close friend says that doing IVF is just ten days of your life. We hard disagree. It is not ten days. It is years of saving for it. The months of tests, of getting dye shot up your fallopian tubes to make sure they're open, of half a dozen blood draws, of being put on thyroid medication even though your thyroid is fine because they want to make sure it "stays fine." Plus all the time and energy you use looking at your patient portal and driving to and from appointments and fielding phone calls about your hormone levels. And then if they find any residue in your fallopian tubes they need to schedule you for a surgery before you can do anything and they cut you open and get rid of the residue to help your chances, or you can go on the hormones and, like my friend Layla, become so sick that you projectile vomit for hours on the bathroom floor. Obviously you lose that cycle so they schedule you for another cycle but since you're out of town during ovulation next month you have to skip that one and do the following month but the following month your partner is out of town so you have to skip that one too so you'll do it a couple months later except that's near your birthday and you don't know if you can take the emotional weight of doing a cycle during your birthday because you know the whole culture about aging and fertility is actual hell on earth. Oh and let's say you do a cycle and it doesn't work and then you're devastated for the rest of your life. If that's just ten days.

How are you supposed to get a test you can't even pronounce the name of? For a year, I put off getting the hysterosalpingography (HSG). The gynecologist puts a catheter of saline up your fallopian tubes to check that they aren't blocked or don't have abnormalities. I am warned that it will hurt and told to take three ibuprofen, but I take a Valium and a Klonopin, both of which I'd bought in Mexico for situations exactly like this. That's the drug addict in me. Kind of like on the HBO series *Hacks* when comedian Meg Stalter barely cuts her finger and is offered Advil and asks for OxyContin.

The test, for someone so squeamish and skittish like me, someone who *clenches*, goes well. There are no cysts, no fibroids, and both fallopian tubes are open. *Your uterus is perfect*, they say. It is shocking. That word again, "perfect." I expected something to be wrong. I think about how I almost didn't get the test. I'd been prepared to spend my life wondering or assuming something was wrong without ever actually knowing if it was or wasn't.

Another day of slinging pants. When people enter I make sure to tell them we have one of each hanging but that there are built-in shelves on the walls where we keep the big stacks from XXS to 4XL. I hold the stacks flat in the palm of my hand, the way one would deliver a pizza.

"How do you go to the bathroom wearing a jumpsuit?"

"You get used to it."

"I can't handle button flies."

"The buttons break in. It's not hard."

Sometimes people ask me if I can tell their size by looking at them. I always say no. It's a trap.

"Thank you for trying," I say to the people who try but don't buy, as they walk out the door.

Whenever I think about my choice to not pursue IVF, I think of being in a booth with two friends about a decade ago. One was describing her anxiety, depression, and insomnia. The other friend said, deadpan, "There are drugs for that."

But IVF seems comparable to getting your MFA. You don't know if you'll get a book or baby out of them, and they likely will put you into debt.

A friend in an MFA program tells me a story. After the program ended, she was in a group chat with her cohort. It was a supportive place where they gave updates about querying agents and book submissions. One day someone announced they sold their book.

A few people responded by being politely excited.

No one spoke in their group chat again.

The 50 percent discount I get at the boutique is always tempting, especially if I shop from the sale rack, which is already marked down by 30 percent. Sometimes at the end of the day I make an unplanned jumpsuit purchase. Emilie Pine writes about this in her book *Notes to Self*, that the longer she didn't get pregnant the more dresses she purchased.

We are allowed to play whatever music we want at the shop, which is unusual. I like queueing up different music for different types of people and age brackets, from oldies to nineties hits. If it's a queer person or couple I'll put on queerish music. Often the partner of the person shopping will comment that they like my music choices. Other times, I hear the person in the dressing room singing along.

I make myself a playlist called Driving for when I go to my blood work, HSG, dildo cam, and follow-up appointments alone. It includes Tori Amos, Elvis Perkins, Ms. White, and the Chicks song "So Hard," which is about the infertility two of them experienced. I listen repeatedly, parked in the Trader Joe's parking lot.

This could be the part of the book where I list everything I've tried: the herbs, the supplements, and everyone's favorite—putting my legs up on the wall after sex. The yoga retreats, the muddy teas and the supplement subscriptions and the probiotics the prebiotics the meditation the books the blah blah blah blah. How I didn't have caffeine for months and spoke to the child when I was driving alone and wrote notes to the spirit in my journal. And it is so boring to fall into that cliché. But it comes from an honest place, because we all know, if we try to get pregnant and don't, someone will tell us why it is our fault and what we did wrong.

"You've handled this really well," one of my friends says.

"You're handling this really well," my mom says.

I shake my head at my mom.

"You don't think you have?"

I think I present as if I have. But they aren't there when the mug or the bowl of soup shatters. They aren't there on the drives to the clinic in the winter and they aren't there taking deep breaths to let the dildo cam glide in. I can pretend I'm handling it well. You get good at what you do.

"Fertility land is full of stories," Esther Perel says on a podcast. "The people with the story of success speak much more loudly than the people it did not work for."

On Reddit, a post in the infertility section says, "Your success stories suck."

The drive to the clinic is ugly as hell, banal, no scenery, and always twenty minutes longer than I want it to be. The Trader Joe's is really the only incentive. There's also a Whole Foods, Barnes & Noble, Sephora. Occasionally I go to the Sephora to replenish my ILIA sunscreen, and to Auntie Anne's for pretzel nuggets I can dip into gross fake cheese on the drive home, licking salt off my fingers. That's the thing about the not-getting-the-baby mindset; you feel you are owed things such as Auntie Anne's pretzel nuggets with fake cheese.

But it's Trader Joe's, seven minutes from the clinic, I find myself in after every blood test and dildo-cam appointment.

Once, when the nurse is giving me a vaginal ultrasound asked what I was up to after my appointment, I was honest with her and told her I'd be going to Trader Joe's. She tells me that's how most women at the fertility clinic respond. Postappointment as I wander around grabbing bacon-flavored dog treats and easy stuff to pack in lunches like string cheese I glance around and wonder which of the other people has just had the dildo cam stuck up them with lube, who else is surviving hell alongside me.

They say dress for the job you want, not the job you have, but I say grocery shop for the family you have, not the family you want.

What time is it? Like, in this book, what time is it? I teach my students about time stamps and cannot bring myself to do them here. I am surprised that the dates of the treatments and medications don't stick vividly in my head. It is all blurry, gray, edges soft. Is it a protective mechanism?

I am asked to interview an author who wrote a novel about post-partum depression. In the same week, I'm asked to blurb a memoir described as being about the creative imperative to have kids/make art. A few days later, I receive an email asking me to blurb a poetry book with motherhood themes, and also a book simply titled *The Book of Mothers*.

After hearing I've been at this for over three years, someone on Reddit suggests I leave the r/TryingForABaby group and head to a different group, a group called r/StillTrying.

Fantasies: Being someone who doesn't want to get pregnant. Being a drug addict. Being a gay man who doesn't want children. Being lethargic and sloppy, drinking bottles and bottles of wine. Being a pill popper like in high school. High on Vicodin. Not having to think about digestion, sugar, alcohol, warm food, room temperature water, caffeine, meditation, antidepressants, yoga, walking, for one day.

For the second year in a row, I attend yoga on Mother's Day, to lift myself from looming depression. At the end of class, the teacher reads a poem called "The Mother Secret" by Sophie Strand. From the second stanza:

> A man can mother his own mother.
> A little girl on the mountain, mothers the summit, the lichen,
> shepherds a salamander across the trail. A woman
> can mother herself, tenderly, by making the coffee
> strong enough, placing the tulips on a butter-circle
> of sun on the windowsill.

Sometimes it's impossible to get through that Arcade Fire song, if it comes on at a bar: "So can you understand / That I want a daughter when I'm still young?"

I google the dude from Arcade Fire to see if he ended up having a daughter while he was still young, and read a bunch of articles about allegations of sexual misconduct against him and how he was canceled.

There are different reactions to ways I greet people when they enter the shop. What comes most naturally to me is "Hi!" but I find it comes off defensive or curt. When I say, "Hi there" or "Hello," people seem more relaxed. "Hi there" seems especially soothing for people. When I'm in one of my extracasual moods, I say, "How's it going?" In the spring and summer I almost always have an iced coffee with me because I'm convinced it makes my personality better even though it probably makes it worse. My mom says it makes me "manic."

Underneath "The Art of Waiting" by Belle Boggs in *Orion* magazine are dozens of comments. One person says that trying to conceive and waiting for it to happen is like waiting for someone who has gone missing each month.

If at first you don't succeed, etc.

Maybe we *can't* do hard things?

Or don't want to?

In yoga, the teacher who years earlier said we were celebrating failure now says, "We love failing. We fail all the time."

My dad says, "You get good at what you do." He tells his guitar students, "If you don't practice, you get really good at not practicing."

One day I have the thought, if you don't get pregnant, you get really good at not getting pregnant.

After the IUI, when the black-aura-inducing Clomid begins to wear off, an article my friend sent me years ago pops into my mind. It was a profile about a fertility-boosting program in a local Hudson Valley magazine. I google until I find it again and reread it, and sign up on the Fertile Heart website.

Julia, the woman who runs the program, is originally from Czechoslovakia and in her seventies. On her first call with me she describes herself as "unpopular," which I like. She calls it a life crisis when the child is summoned and does not come. She also reframes the crisis as an opportunity. I am at the point where if I stay a victim I'd have a miserable life, so thinking of it as an opportunity resonates with me. Her philosophy isn't about conceiving naturally—it's about opening your heart to whatever path becomes right for you: adoption, surrogacy, being child-free. She isn't anti-IVF, but she also doesn't see it as the only way.

She calls her meetings Visionary Support Circles. The meetings are unwieldy, unpredictable, and occasionally inappropriate. Sometimes there are six of us, sometimes twenty.

She says that when the child is summoned and doesn't come, it's because the mother hasn't yet been born.

The biopsy for endometriosis is more painful than any of the other tests. More than the dildo cam, which doesn't hurt at all, and even more than the HSG. I yell "fuck" a few times and they tell me that is fine. In the following weeks, I forget all about the biopsy and whenever I remember my heart does a little flutter, thinking I could be called with news at any minute. I am so excited that I might have endometriosis—that there would be a reason for everything.

I miss the days my heart would flutter over crushes or exes or meeting someone for sex instead of endometriosis biopsies.

When they call with the results, I'm disappointed and still unexplained.

In Paris for a destination writing retreat where I am teaching, the thought of pregnancy goes away. Why? The wine, the cheese? I don't eat cured meats not because of pregnancy but because I don't like them. I eat escargot and pâté and baguettes and Comté. There are zero thoughts of too much caffeine or alcohol and I only occasionally see a stroller.

On the train into the Black Forest, Germany, the thoughts creep in loudly again. I spend the weekend with a friend but say nothing about it, drink whiskey, eat bratwursts and big buttered pretzels.

B is on tour in Australia. We aren't communicating much, and I am slightly proud of how strong our relationship is. We are an unconventional traveling-artist couple and can withstand these frequent and separate work trips. We do send emails every evening, with rundowns of our days.

One night on the air mattress I have a dream about going to see a gynecologist. He is someone I saw in real life years ago; in the dream, he shows me a computer screen just as he did in real life. He points to photographs of my fallopian tubes and uterus and strongly suggests that I do IVF. He tells me that one round would be around $2,560 and the second round would be three thousand dollars. He says something about getting those prices through health insurance and Groupon. I am a little intrigued since I know the prices for IVF range from twenty thousand to thirty thousand dollars per round, but I still firmly tell him no; I tell him my mind was made up years ago.

You aren't listening to me, I say. Stop asking! Then I wake up.

In a church in the Black Forest, there is hand sanitizer in one dispenser and holy water in another dispenser. My friend mixes them up, so we bless ourselves with hand sanitizer.

The Fertile Heart Visionary Support Circles give me a whole new vocabulary. Julia uses the term "holy human loaf" instead of "body." Sometimes she makes us look up to the sky or ceiling and wave to the "circle of babies."

"We are not victims, we are adventurers," she says at the end of one call. "We are fertile adventurers. There is no such thing as failure in this neighborhood," she says.

It feels so good to laugh, but she is not trying to be funny.

Another day, another acupuncturist, since the other one is on maternity leave. This one is walking distance from my apartment. When I describe my situation to him from a plastic folding chair, he asks me, "Any theories?"

Theories: Body glitter and its toxins from the nineties. Karma for every lipstick and shirt I stole, the people I fucked, the drugs up the nose, for texting and driving. Using curly-hair products containing phthalates for probably ten years before anyone talked about ingredients. Self-tanner, tanning beds, spray tans, getting hair balayage. My MacBook Air hot on my lap frying my eggs. Caffeine. The chemicals in receipts. Wine. Tequila. Kratom. Age. My marriage wasn't ready. Make plans, God laughs, etc. Some cysts and polyps they managed not to see during the test. Endometriosis they didn't find with the test. I'm supposed to write this book instead. God wants me to be forty. I'm blocking conception because of something spiritually. I don't do enough cardio. Antidepressants. Never had Reiki. Don't want it badly enough. Want it too badly. The world is waiting to do something cruel to me, like get me pregnant the year one of my parents dies. Bathing in fragrance because I didn't know it was an endocrine disruptor.

Theories: none.

Theories. How much time do you have?

What I told him: how I'm cold all the time.

Now that I've shopped so much at Trader Joe's, every other grocery store seems expensive and boring. They don't get your mind off infertility the way Trader Joe's does, with its disgusting pumpkin ice cream and chocolate hummus and cheap workhorse skin care.

After a few months' break of trying and treatments, it is time again. During the first IUI, I'd been prescribed a thyroid medication, even though my thyroid is in normal range. It was to keep it there. I'd stopped taking the medication when I stopped trying for the summer. I knew if I called the clinic and asked if I should begin taking it again, they'd tell me I have to go in for blood work. This is calculated on my part, because if they tell me I need to go in for blood work, I can go to Trader Joe's for rose water toner and garlic-stuffed olives and dried mango.

It works; they ask me to come on Tuesday at 8:00 a.m.

When I pick up the letrozole prescription, the pharmacist calls me "love." It's the best part of my day.

Letrozole does the same thing as Clomid: it makes you grow extra eggs, but without the side effects, they tell me. I wonder why they would start me on the one with negative side effects, but no one seems to have answers for my questions.

The second IUI doesn't get me pregnant either. B is out of town when I get the phone. It's breezy and sunny and springy out and I'm taking a hot-girl walk wearing a Stevie Nicks T-shirt. I'm not even shocked. I keep walking, blasting King Princess and Mitski and I don't die. Instead I "go home and boil noodles, like every grieving mother everywhere," as Catherine Newman writes in her novel *Sandwich*.

We have the routine down by the third IUI. B jerks off into a cup in his music studio while I wait in the car. On the drive, I hold the cup of sperm between my legs because they instruct you to keep it warm. We talk about how to continue doing IUIs since he is leaving for tour soon. I am always thinking ahead in six-month chunks. We agree to look into how much it costs to freeze-sperm.

The sperm needs to be dropped off an hour earlier to be washed— they weed out weaker sperm so you're only left with the most motile ones—so we go out to breakfast. Back at the clinic, only I go in, as partners aren't allowed even in the waiting room, some kind of postpandemic rule. I put my feet in the stirrups. I always wear cozy and warm socks. The nurse brings in a sheet of paper she calls a "report card" for the sperm. They want at least five million for a good chance. We have way more than that, she says. She inserts it and it's over and she leaves the room.

In *The Argonauts*, Maggie Nelson writes about bringing herself to orgasm at her IUI while her partner, Harry Dodge, holds her—less for romance and more because science says it helps the odds. But I just lay there by myself, breathing.

When I get the call, I'm sitting on the couch. B is on tour. I don't flinch. I'm used to not getting pregnant. It's my normal, resting state.

With the book *Taking Charge of Your Fertility* in my arms, I walk to the free library and put it on the shelf. Let someone else take charge of their fertility.

I sell the Ava bracelet fertility tracker I purchased for three hundred dollars on my credit card a year prior to someone on Reddit. Wait, I don't sell it, I give it away for free. Even though the Ava company promises they'll give you your money back if you're not pregnant within a year, I can't imagine going through with a return like that. What would I say to customer service? Was I so young and naive I thought a bracelet would get me pregnant? You bet.

In *The Room Lit by Roses* Carole Maso writes:

> The child I had spent years writing about in my *Bay of Angels* notebooks. When I look back I see that she is there in one way or another in many, many guises. My writing life, as always, so much further ahead of my conscious, rational mind. How had I been so blind? There she was at the periphery of every page, waiting, begging at the edge of language, calling my name. But I did not, could not recognize her—until it was very nearly too late.

I have written about unborn children in my published books and my journals. In my first book, published when I was twenty-six, I compared myself to Anne Lamott, wrote that I'd felt sorry in advance for the son I would have, because I'd be writing about him all the time, as Lamott did in her book *Operating Instructions*.

When I read from that book the audience laughed and I laughed with them. Because obviously this would be true! Of course I'd have kids. I remember where I was standing, who was in my line of vision, what I was wearing when I read that line.

A few years before any real trying, I received some mail from my insurance company telling me infertility treatment was now covered: up to three IUIs and basic testing. At the time, I still thought I'd get pregnant perfectly accidentally, but there was still some glimmer of relief, as if on some level of consciousness I knew I was going to use it. I left it in a corner of my desk.

After one of the IUIs (Which? Who knows? Who cares?) I am home putting groceries away and get a call from my insurance. They say they'd heard I am pregnant. My breath stops. For a second, I actually think my insurance company, UnitedHealthcare, is calling to break the news that I'm pregnant, because the fertility clinic has gotten the positive test and accidentally told my insurance company before telling me.

"We heard you're pregnant," they say. They say that.

I let them know that I could be pregnant but wouldn't know for another week, because I am not Phoebe on *Friends*.

They say to call them back if I am pregnant. We don't speak again.

I drink wine with the owner of the boutique. After two glasses of sauvignon blanc, I have the idea that she should put LIFE CHANGING PANTS on the new tote bags she's creating. The slogan starts so many conversations, I tell her. We talk about the jumpsuits for the following spring, whether they should be pink or purple.

Twice a year, I get a "clothing benefit" where I'm allowed to choose two items from the shop. I tell the owner I'll lock up fifteen minutes after closing time so I can try on pants and jumpsuits. It actually takes me an hour and fifteen minutes. I use all the techniques I tell the customers to use. I put my shoes on to see how the pants will look in real life. I sit down to feel if they're too tight. I leave with a new jumpsuit and evergreen pants.

A few weeks later, I am reading an interview with a parenting expert, and she writes how having a child is "profoundly life-changing." But apparently, so are curve-friendly, well-made, 98 percent cotton and 2 percent spandex, size-inclusive pants.

Someone somewhere brings to my attention that you can go to Prague and do IVF for $2,500. I join a Facebook group called IVF in Prague and research dozens of fertility clinics there. The tone of their emails back to me is so different from the ones in the United States. They call me by name, ask me how I am, and seem to mean it. They use smiley emojis at the ends of their emails. When they take a while to respond, they apologize and say it's because they got the flu. B and I agree this might be the golden ticket, in our budget—plus we get to see Prague! But it's impossible to schedule, and when we bring the issue to therapy, B makes it clear he's prioritizing his tour. He wants to come just for the days he'd need to provide sperm. Being alone in a foreign country on hormonal medication doesn't seem wise for me, so the idea never comes to fruition.

On a thick July night, my dad and I are drinking wine on my porch with his friend. A summer earlier, her husband passed away. She is talking this night about moving on, about dating. She's moved into a new house, and many of the logistics of his passing are done.

"I don't know." She shrugs. "What do I do now?"

"Lean forward and run down the hill," my dad responds.

I thought it sounded like a profound life mantra and maybe the title of a novel. His friend says it sounds like a fiftieth-birthday Hallmark card.

My friend's son asks me, "What's something everyone in the world has in common?"

"What?"

"They all have a biological mother."

I have to drive to urgent care for a hangnail that has gotten infected. In the waiting room the television plays health facts every thirty seconds. Then the urgent care slogan shows up: *We can handle anything life throws your way.*

Outside the window by my desk there is a bird's nest and occasionally I can hear the mother feeding her babies. If I were a different kind of writer, I'd make this bird's nest a motif, a metaphor, and return to it every twenty pages or so. But I don't feel like it.

Outside my window, a squirrel curls in a tree. A cat lies on the roof in the sun.

There is a sadistic pleasure I get from telling people they are wrong at the boutique. When they ask if we only have wide-leg pants and I get to say No. When they ask if we have a bathroom and I get to say No. When they ask if we have change for a dollar for the parking meter and I get to say No. When they ask if we are open on Monday. When they ask if we are open on Tuesday. When they ask if we are open on Wednesday. When they ask if I'm about to close. When they ask, disappointed and surprised, standing at the sale rack, if the price on the tag is the sale price and I get to say Yes.

The psychiatrist Phil Stutz says that one of the tools of life is accepting you will always be dealing with "pain, uncertainty, and constant work."

My shoulders relax after hearing that. So this isn't a phase. This will be life.

One night in a black mood, I say to my friend Mia, "In ten years I'll either be in an open marriage or divorced."

Later we are walking in the East Village talking about crushes and pining. She says something like, "Well, you're like married and shit," implying I don't get it.

"You can still be married and pine," I say.

"Oh, word?" She glances quickly over at me.

Over drinks with another friend she says, "I always forget you're married."

"Yeah, because I don't *seem* married," I say.

At three o'clock in the afternoon I go for a glass of wine with my mom, because I have a fun mom. I am in an optimistic place and say to her that in some ways the longer this goes on, the easier it gets. It is hard to explain. Some might say it is unexplained.

"I just don't want you to be heartbroken," she says.

"Oh, well *of course* I'm heartbroken!" I say dismissively and her face falls.

A man opens the door and asks, "Do you like art?" It is a complicated question, since I do in fact like art but I also know he is going to try to sell me something that I don't want. I resent him for putting me in the position of having to say firmly, No, I don't like art.

A man walks by the shop and I hear him say, "Every time I walk by that sign, I . . ." Since he is in motion, I didn't get to hear the end of his sentence.

I am writing feedback for a student: "This is so fertile and juicy . . ." Then I delete it. Ew.

One afternoon, day one of my menstrual cycle, it is deceivingly warm outside, the fifth day of spring. I walk into a grocery store in a red barn where I need nothing and buy orange-creamsicle French ice cream, feng shui spray, and two hard seltzers. It is a chaotic purchase, even for me. I consider all the money I don't spend on diapers. The cashier tells me it is forty-five dollars, and I do my best not to flinch. I walk home, opening the pint of ice cream and eating it with my teeth.

One late night I scour the internet for people who deeply desire a child but have decided IVF is not for them. We are a small group. One person says the process around IVF makes her body feel broken. You're constantly told it isn't working properly, it isn't doing the thing it should be doing naturally, you don't have enough eggs, maybe you have endometriosis, a messed-up uterus, fallopian tubes, you're too old, unlucky.

She explains that she'd rather do things that make her body feel whole and intact, activities like dancing, hiking, swimming, walking, cooking. This comment rearranges my whole brain.

I drive to Burlington, Vermont, for a two-hour appointment with a naturopath and pay three hundred dollars for it, the most I've ever spent on one appointment. She tells me that maitake mushrooms do the same thing that Clomid does.

Why didn't I just lie to people about trying? I wish lying came more easily to me. Why didn't I tell people I was ambivalent, conflicted— I was an artist!—and that I was doing the whole trying and not preventing? Why did I have to say something years ago?

Because I thought it would go like this: I'd tell people I was trying, and six months later I'd be pregnant, and everyone would see that I get what I want when I want it.

Did I think trying to become pregnant made me *interesting*?

Writing publicly is so embarrassing. But someone's gotta do it. In her book *The Buddhist*, Dodie Bellamy makes the case for more operatic grand public suffering in writing. I'd read the book back in 2013 and it was a major influence.

"I really took that notion and ran with it," I say to Mia.

"Straight into a career," she responds.

On my days off I wear skinny jeans because to work I only wear wide legs. I'm walking back from the DMV and run into Reggo washing the windows of a vintage-clothing store. He washes the windows of the pants store biweekly too. He does the whole strip of shops, which all contain items no one needs, and even includes a make-your-own-candle bar.

I've only ever seen him in a mask, but you can tell by his eyes he is always smiling. He brings me mango occasionally, sometimes lychee, and jalapeño peppers. He stays to talk longer than most people would, and I know that his wife thinks the peppers are too spicy and that he can't drink cow's milk. He likes mixing up English and Spanish and when he leaves he does a handshake or a fist bump or elbow pump or high five.

When I ask him how he is, he says he ended up in the hospital. He mimics crying, rubbing his eyes, and tells me he's been crying for five months. "In the streets, at my home," he says. "Depression," he says.

If someone had asked me if I knew Reggo the window washer, I would have said, yes, the guy that's always happy. Now, whenever I see him, he says "good friend" to me when he waves goodbye.

For some reason, I stop running or hiding or cowering from pregnant people. I embrace them when they come into the store. I recommend the 100 percent cotton button-down jumpsuits for breastfeeding. I know exactly which overalls and jumpsuits are stretchiest and will work for a few more months as they grow. One day I sell two pregnant customers jumpsuits, one after the other.

An Aldi grocery shop opens up and is a four-minute drive from my apartment. It's not quite Trader Joe's but it is fantastic in its own right. This complicates things, because I don't need an excuse to go to the fertility clinic anymore as an excuse to go to Trader Joe's, and if I'm not driving to Trader Joe's, do I really want a child at all?

ACT III

I began to understand what a story is. It's a manipulation.
A way of containing unmanageable chaos.

—*Sarah Manguso,* Liars

Quick question: If the writer is writing a book about trying to get pregnant for a little over two years, from the comfort of her closet office in the apartment she lives in with her husband, and the book was sold as a book about trying to get pregnant, in the circumstance she was in, which was under a roof with her husband and his sperm, and then the writer divorces him and it affects the concept of her book, does she owe it to the reader to be included?

Celebrities Who've Announced Their Divorces While I've Been Trying

Emily Ratajkowski
Miranda July
Shakira
Sophia Bush
Katie Holmes
Britney Spears
Ariana Grande
Jennifer Lopez
Kim Kardashian
Sara Ramirez
Busy Philipps

Celebrities Who've Come Out as Gay While I've Been Trying

Reneé Rapp
Sophia Bush
Chappell Roan
Rebel Wilson
Jerrod Carmichael
Julia Fox

On my thirty-seventh birthday in early April, B was on tour and barely wished me a happy birthday, so I asked him what was up. Over the phone, he continued to comfortably lie that it was "nothing," but I wouldn't let it go. I felt sick and was shaking. An hour later he admitted to getting hand jobs at massage parlors.

A week later it was blow jobs at massage parlors.

I kept pushing.

He added nuru massages.

On May 1, after an intense argument, he finally admitted that he saw one prostitute, during tour in Europe in one of the red-light districts, I walked to work at the pants store. The second I got there, I downloaded a dating app and Zillow, Trulia, and StreetEasy. Fifteen minutes later he burst through the door and said he'd spent thousands of dollars on prostitutes over the last two years.

He told me he had a problem, and that he might write a book about it "to help other men," and then he left, shutting the door behind him.

I don't remember selling any pants that day.

When I got home from the shop I walked over to the buckets in my writing closet, filled with gruesome yellow-and-orange water. I tried throwing them on him but I mostly missed. "Not the water!" I think he yelled. He later told people I attacked him.

Welp, my life blew up, I text a friend.

Our mutual friend gets B to a medical clinic and when I call him there he is stripped down to a hospital gown and I'm house-sitting in New Orleans. They put me on hold and the music is "I'll Make Love to You" by Boyz II Men and I laugh. He starts crying when he hears my voice. After a couple of weeks at the clinic his family pays for him to attend a thirty-day sex-addiction center called Seeking Integrity.

"Maybe the unexplained is now explained," my stepdaughter says.

How does a book about irresolution end? What is the reader owed? What is the writer owed?

Will the writer still be trying to get pregnant when she becomes single?

Will the voice change? The structure? Tone? Is this even allowed in a book if you didn't know it was the book you were writing?

Should the writer continue the book in the same style, using fragments and notes? Or should she change the style to signify the seismic shift?

Should she break the fourth wall, perhaps putting the problem into the work itself?

Which personal details should she omit?

How should she queer the narrative? What does that even mean?

Is it relevant that the writer's queer novella went out of print the same years she was married to a man?

If you're writing about your life in real time, are you inherently fucked?

I ask B for a list of the dates when this all happened. The dates correspond with our wedding anniversaries, my book tour, significant birthdays.

One evening before I did a reading in the East Village, I'd called him in Geneva, Switzerland. He'd sounded odd and slow, and there were typos in all his text messages. My body buzzed with anxiety. I asked him what was going on and he said he'd smoked weed, something he wasn't supposed to be doing because it lowers sperm count.

"Oh honey, that's fine!" I'd said. Now he admits he'd done cocaine, drank copious whiskey, and had not one, not two, but three sex workers to his hotel room that night. He'd sent me an email that same night about how grateful he was for me, how he was the luckiest man in the world, what an amazing wife and stepmom I was.

I remember that I'd turned down an editor asking me to be in an anthology called *I Feel Love: Notes on Queer Joy.* I didn't have anything for it, I'd told her.

B tries to repair, leaving vases of roses, writing long emails, begging and pleading and crying on the floor in the corner. He sends cards, one, confusingly, with one-hundred dollars cash inside. He says he will do anything to fight for this relationship, for his reputation. He will do absolutely anything to fight for me, for us, for our family, he says. Then he gives up.

I'm on a flight to New Orleans and there is buzzing in my chest and time speeds up and I'm either flying or drowning or numbing and the buzzing won't go away so I drink sauvignon blanc and oh my god I lost my life and I lost my family my friend flies straight to my door and we drink wine and we drink coffee after coffee after coffee even though it makes the buzzing worse it's a simple pleasure and I need a reason to get up and he has taken so much from me I won't let him take away coffee plus it's spring the best season for cold brew and iced coffee and what is spring into summer without that I can't eat until it's so late in the day and I get tacos and beer even though I don't drink beer it's what they sell at Rosalita's taco shop and I can't think of what to order I won't be able to think of what food to order for the next three even four even five months after all those months of cook-ing and eating only warm fertility food now I put anything into my body the cold brew Sancerre the tacos and I walk with my dad along the Mississippi River every day and everyone else is on Planet Earth and I'm on Planet Divorce and Planet Prostitute and I get burned from the sun and my dad looks distraught when I tell him what hap-pened he puts his hands over his face and we get Thai food and see the *Are You There, God? It's Me, Margaret.* movie and I say *I'm sorry I'm here while I'm in crisis* and he says *If you're in crisis it is exactly when you better be here* and it's so kind I cry and everyone is worried about me sleeping and eating and my mom mails trazodone to my dad's and I fly home to my mom's because I don't have a home anymore so from my dad's I go to my mom's just like when I was a teenager and I'm a child of divorce going through my own divorce and I lie in the ham-mock and lie on the deck and lie on the sunporch and we talk and we talk and we talk and watch *Abbott Elementary* and walk in the woods and the mornings are still bad and at one point she says *Mornings are hard for you aren't they* and she sits next to me on the couch and gives me coffee and I lie in the sun and I walk in the woods and my uncle sends me a note and my aunt sends me money and my other aunt sends me a cookbook and money and my other aunt sends me a post-card and my other aunt sends me an email and my other aunt sends me another cookbook because they want to help me they feel help-less no one knows what to do and I have lunch with my editor and when I tell her she puts her hands over her face the same way my dad did and I call my childhood friends and I call my newer friends and I pace up and down my mom's driveway and they listen and I call my newer friends and they listen and I can't listen to Lana Del Rey any-more even though she's the only thing I want to listen to and I send mean texts I unblock I block I unblock and I get on Tinder and I'm at a Marriott in Chelsea with a person who carries a strap-on in her tote bag and then I'm packing and finding all the wedding cards we were sent and my friends help me move into a studio and they hang up my art and make sure I have plants and cleaning supplies and sage and we go out to dinner after and the moving is so fun, so joyous, a party, and I love my new deck and flowers and windows and I go to Planned Parenthood for STD testing and then I'm in a Marriott again and having orgasms and watching her sleep and she's making me laugh and fucking me on the sink on the desk we sleep holding each other we crack each other up we banter we piss each other off we're both sensitive and guarded as fuck we sleep in our necklaces and she comes to my new studio apartment where there are zero memories she sees my art and she looks at all the books on my shelves while saying *Stop tryna date me* I say *Stop tryna date me I'm in the middle of a divorce* we kiss and kiss and kiss and send each other songs we send each other photos we sleep until noon and then I'm flying to Paris for teaching and still drinking wine still not knowing what kind of food to order and eating only cherries and yogurt even though everyone is texting me to eat a chocolate croissant for them or eat a banana-and-Nutella crepe for them or eat a croque monsieur for them but I don't and I discover polyamory and for a month text every single day with Riley and we have phone sex while I'm in my bed at an Airbnb in Montmartre when it's 5:00 a.m. my time and 11:00 p.m. her time and we both come hard and the sun comes up and I think about sperm donors I think about asking friends for sperm I think about the past six years and refuse to have the thought "my most fertile years wasted" because I hate when people say that and I keep moving forward and I buy *The Woman Destroyed* by Simone de Beauvoir at the Abbey Bookshop in the Latin Quarter to be basic and I drink so much coffee for something to do something to live for and I can't handle silence anymore I listen to audiobooks about divorce I listen to comedians I listen to podcasts I listen to music and Lana Del Rey makes me too unhinged but it's all I want and I'm already unhinged and I show up at my friend's house hyperventilating in a sweatshirt and he says, *I got you, come here* and he calls me every day every single fucking morning of May and June and July and a new level of friendship is unlocked and we log hundreds and hundreds maybe thousands of hours on the phone and now I understand what intimacy actually is he reminds me I am loved and that my agency had been taken away but now my agency is back

A friend texts: *I'm thinking of you and you will get glimpses of how good life will be once it is less painful. Remember who you are! Strong, intelligent, loving! You are still in shock but you will find peace.*

I'm a special kind of tired, I write back. *But where I'm housesitting has an outdoor shower.*

My stepdaughter hands me a folded three-page letter she wrote in pencil on lined school paper. *You will go on to have a great family with a great person*, she writes. *And I will ALWAYS be with you, because I will always be your stepdaughter. And you will always be my stepmom!* She writes we should read a Judy Blume book together. She writes that these weeks have been the longest time she hasn't seen me in "maybe ever." She writes, *I'm honestly happy for you.*

She writes that if I'm ever really mad, I should listen to the song, "Cell Block Tango." *I have been, and it's pretty fun*, she writes, adding (*Just don't actually kill anyone* ☺) in parentheses. She adds a p.s. telling me she's been listening to the song "White Dress" by Lana Del Rey. She ends the letter with *YOU WILL ALWAYS BE MY STEPMOM* in all caps, and a p.p.s. where she has drawn seven hearts.

JD says, "I'll set up your apartment and make it look like you've lived there for months," and then he does. Marty takes me to Lowe's where we buy ferns and a yellow rosebush. After potting flowers all day, he takes a photo of me on my deck, in Converse surrounded by the ferns and roses.

"You look hot and *gay*," Hannah says about my deck-and-ferns photo, and I post it to Hinge.

Hannah has always been gay but married a man, and is convinced some of us who are openly queer or queer leaning marry men because "it's biological. We think it will be an easy way to have kids."

She tells me a memory: after she became pregnant with her second child, she said to her sister, "I never have to have sex with a man again!" She'd played it as a joke; she knew it wasn't.

The first morning on my deck, writing in my journal, it is as though I was back from a detour. Like I'd gotten sidetracked and now was back to my life.

"You never fully fused," my therapist says about B and me.

Three and a half weeks after moving into my new apartment, my mom is over for dinner on the deck and we see a double rainbow.

My stepdaughter comes over after school and we have Gouda and garlic-stuffed olives on the deck. She runs down the hill in the yard, talks about sledding there in the winter. "At least the utilities here work!" she says. When I ask what she means she says the place we used to live was "falling apart and janky."

When she turns thirteen a week later in June, I have a birthday party for her and she blows out her cake candles at my kitchen counter. She's wearing my hand-me-down Everlane jeans, Madewell blouse, and heels from Poshmark. Before the party, we sang the Billie Eilish song, "when the party's over" in a community-choir concert together. Her dad isn't there, still Seeking Integrity.

I don't yet know that this is the last time I will be allowed to see her, that she will be instructed to have no contact with me for the unforeseeable future.

Everyone reminds me I have my writing, like it's a consolation for the grief.

"You have six months," JD says.

"Six months for what?" I ask.

"To be extravagantly crazy," he responds.

It's June it's pride and I ride the train on a Sunday to New York City with a rainbow bracelet on my wrist for a first date with Riley. I wear sneakers and a leather jacket and red dress. "Is it even a date if someone doesn't wear a leather jacket?" she says. She wears a mustard cashmere sweater. It's the first time in six years I don't have to tell anyone where I am. We meet in Madison Square Park where she's sitting on a bench. She later told me she intentionally chose that bench. "I wanted to see you before you could see me," she said. *We can catch the sunset*, she'd texted in advance. But we don't.

Instead, we make out in the nearly pitch-black booth in a speakeasy and melt into each other. I pull her two silver chains toward me. Her fingers find my tights. When we are gathering our tote bags to leave—mine *The New Yorker*, hers Dr. Martens—I say: "Sometimes I wonder if I was mostly with him because of the easy access to sperm."

"That's something I'll never need," she says.

We hold hands on the way to Walgreens for gum and cash, and on the way to the Arlo NoMad bathroom to make out, on the way to Vin Sur Vingt Wine Bar, on the way to the Marriott, on the way to my hotel bed.

How am I holding hands with a stranger? Four weeks ago I was married with a dog and a car and fridge full of food and ovulation and pregnancy tests. But is she really any more a stranger than the person I was married to?

All the thoughts that consumed me of eating only warm food, of drinking room temperature water, are gone. My body is mine again. It is not at the mercy of doctors or B's tour schedule or ovulation or Clomid or letrozole or a period app or fertility app or Ava bracelet or the dildo cam or metal stirrups or a waiting room or calendar or phone call.

My texts stop autocorrecting to "infertility" and "IVF." One day I am trying to describe medicine and forget the word letrozole.

However I survive this is okay is what I tell myself after reading it in Leslie Jamison's book *Splinters*.

People are afraid to ask me how I am. When they tentatively say, "How are you?" they look scared. And they should be.

How is it that now, stopping fertility treatments, being four years older than I was when I began trying, that I feel so much more confident I will have a child? The possibilities feel endless now. It feels like there is a creativity to the whole thing that was lacking before. There is optimism. I remember the part in *The Argonauts* where donor sperm from Maggie Nelson's friend sat in a glass jar that was once Newman's Own salsa. And the part in *Knocking Myself Up* by Michelle Tea where she has a bunch of friends over and her girlfriend inseminates her with a drag queen's sperm.

In her book *Love Me Tender*, Constance Debré explains her getting-younger-when-getting-gayer theory:

> You gain ten years, easy, when you become gay. Everyone knows that. Dorian Gray effect guaranteed. I say this for the benefit of straight mothers everywhere. They're often quite depressed about aging. There's a simple solution. Just so they know. You could say at twenty I was actually forty and today I'm twenty. That's what people tell me. They say I'm living my teenage years now.

A friend just under thirty years old falls madly in love with a woman at a wedding and they spend months flying back and forth between California and New York to see each other. One night at a bar in the East Village, she and I are talking about pregnancy and fertility testing. She knows I want children and I know she is conflicted. She tells me her girlfriend who is over forty is just now considering her fertility. She says: "Lesbians who have always been lesbians have very little conception of how women get pregnant. She's thinking about freezing her eggs, an idea that seems to have no urgency to her. Meanwhile every straight girl I know under the age of thirty-two has already frozen their eggs and I'd had two abortions and a miscarriage by age twenty-nine."

Even if lesbians and gay people start the process later, they really have to try. In a 2018 essay, Katie Heaney writes, "As a queer woman, I can't afford to be ambivalent about motherhood." In her book *Inconceivable*, Valerie Bauman writes,

> A unique grief can occur with some lesbian partners because they cannot—at least where science is currently—have a baby that shares both of their DNA. A lesbian couple will never "accidentally" get pregnant or be able to take the advice "stop trying so hard" and "let things happen." Every step of the way must be paved with intention and grueling effort.

Was it that my approach toward getting pregnant, the intention and grueling effort, helped my queerness resurface? Had I been approaching getting pregnant like a queer person?

———

I ask my dad the same thing his friend did that July night on the porch. A version of, *Now what? What do I do?*

"Lean forward and run down the hill," he repeats. I ask him if this is because of my age. Like I've been climbing the hill and now in my late thirties I'm going down.

"No," he says. "It's like, make a decision and just do it. Stop thinking about should I or shouldn't I, and just act."

Were the sperm swimming away from me the whole time?

Was my body protecting me?

The body keeps the score, etc.

The body remembers, etc.

The body rejects the sperm, etc.

Is my body that wise?

Some delays are protection.

When I pitched this book to my editor, I stressed that I wanted the book to be a body floating in space. I said, at the end of the day, your partner, husband, mother, doctor, best friend cannot get pregnant for you, nor are the stakes as high for them.

In her essay "New Life," Kate Osterloh writes: "Giving birth, like dying, is something you do alone—plugged into machines, tape on your arm, acid burning your throat. Your lover, asleep nearby, might as well be in another state."

Writing and trying to conceive are two more activities you do alone.

My editor took my pitch and proposal and pages into her meeting and when she gave me feedback over the phone she told me one of her colleagues had questions about the context. "Is she trying to become a single mom?" her colleague asked.

No, she wasn't. But give her a couple of months.

I see, now, that my writing knew something before I did.

I'd also made the decision to omit being a stepmom from the book. I thought it would distract from the zoomed-in feeling of "trying."

It is only now, the day I am handing in the book, my final chance, that I change my mind. At the last second, before I'm not allowed to make any more changes, I add her. She cannot, will not, be erased from my life. Or my book.

What could I say about being a stepmom?

That loving her since she'd been six was the simplest, easiest love I've ever experienced.

That I didn't know losing her this way was even a possibility.

That language for the psychic pain of it fails me—but I still keep writing.

There's no card for Holy Shit! You Lost Your Stepdaughter, Your Favorite Person in the World. Holy Shit! Your Life Blew Up. And So Did Hers. Holy Shit! Hope You're Ready to Always Be Actively Grieving. Holy Shit! One Morning You're Packing Lunch and Running to the School Bus and the Next, Your Texts Don't Deliver!

Postdivorce, the world is vivid. Music has more depth. There's a reason they call it a fog lifting. I blare Mitski and MUNA and dance. The sky and greenery are bright. Though I am full of rage I am equally full of relief. As if the whole being-married-to-a-man thing was cosplay. As if I got married to a man just to make sure I definitely didn't want to be married to a man. Try everything once!

There are no more drives to Albany and Trader Joe's. I'd always hated that ugly and bleak drive and now I don't have to go. Actually, now I couldn't go if I wanted to. We only have two Ubers here, and it seems bizarre to take an Uber to a fertility clinic, even though people probably do it all the time in other cities. But I live in a more rural area, and I don't want to spend more than two hundred dollars on a fifty-minute Uber just to get the dildo cam.

This is a controversial opinion: Having your life blow up is somewhat fun. It means you're in reality all the time. Friends come into focus. Writing comes into focus. Dormant desires come into focus. Complacency, contentment, is gone. It's like being a child again, like being in a foreign country, like being reborn.

Suddenly I can create my living space, my days, my relationships exactly the way I want to. What would life be? Whom would I meet? How would I want to spend my time? I haven't felt this free since I was twenty circa 2006—with a mattress on the floor in Brooklyn.

The first week of May 2023, I lost a husband, an apartment, a step-child, a dog, and a car.

Women talk about having it all. Try having nothing!

Are you okay, a friend texts me.

Nope but I function, I write back immediately, which feels like the most honest response I've ever given, to anyone, to anything, ever.

It occurs to me later how high functioning I look on the outside. I'm the lowest high-functioning person you'll ever meet. Or the highest low-functioning person.

I'm walking with a friend in the Latin Quarter in Paris and she talks about her frozen shoulder. It reminds me of seven years ago, when I was at a writing residency and one morning went to a yoga class with another writer. I was twenty-eight, she was maybe forty, and she told me she had a frozen shoulder. When I asked her what caused it she simply said, "Divorce."

Paris gobbles a day like nothing I've ever seen. It's always noon, then easily 10:00 p.m., then two in the morning. After a few days, I stopped resisting it. I go to a bar called Résistance with my aunt and cousin and mom and we dance in the basement to Dire Straits and French pop and it is hours of unfettered joy.

"It seems like there's more of you now," JD says.

Hannah, who met me a few months before my marriage ended, says I was more subdued then. "That was the only time I've ever heard you have a negative framework on your life," she says.

Coming out of a spa where I got a massage I see a sign. NEW! WE OFFER WIFE DAY CARE. DROP OFF YOUR WIFE WHILE YOU GOLF OR HAVE A BEER OR ALONE TIME.

I rejoice as I walk away, ecstatic to not live in the world where a sign like this means anything. I am not a wife! My membership in that world has ceased.

And I never have to be one again!

I've never dated anyone even a year younger than me before and Riley is six. She calls me "old lady" while we are walking up the hill from the Amtrak station. We never get coffee because she "hates coffee shops, especially new ones." Riley also hates the way I hold my wineglass and how I cross the street in the middle of the road. I hate that she can't make plans more than two hours in advance. But she loves my book collection, and that I give her books, and I love the way I lose all sense of space and time when she kisses my ribs. She is the first person in my new apartment, on my new deck, in my new bed, new sheets. I may not have fully fused with my ex-husband, but with Riley I do fuse, psychologically and energetically. She texts *bed?* at the exact time I get in bed, and *train?* at the moment I sit on the train. Before any literary event I have, she asks what I'll be reading.

My friend wonders why I have such a soft spot for her, then muses out loud, "It's the fallacy of the first."

For hours, I'm in Ridgewood in her bed with gray sheets, the M train out the window becoming a soundtrack. She puts on her playlist while we have a candle burning. She uses the same playlist for all the people she sleeps with. I don't care. Life has made you nihilistic, a friend tells me. You don't believe in love, she says. She's wrong, though. I do believe in love, just not in the same way I used to.

My life feels like *Sliding Doors* when I'm with Riley—I so easily could have not been here. How did I get here? How was I suddenly learning someone else's pizza preferences and the names of their plants and their sleeping style? In her sleep she made the noise of scratching her throat the same way my childhood friend did. We drank sour beers and listened to records, and sometimes I'd hit her blunt. What happened to vacuuming and meal prep? How was I here now, listening to the M train screech, talking about how many times we'd each been in love, listening to "Sittin' Up in My Room" by Brandy? I lend her a book about your brain being on music and another about polyamory. She gives me a half-eaten psilocybin chocolate bar and podcast microphones she doesn't use anymore.

We sometimes sleep until 11:00 a.m. holding each other and when I'd get home, she'd text, *Tell me you miss me.* She has to give a wedding speech and I ask her if she wants help writing it.

"Yeah, I hate writing long-form. I hate writing in general," she says. "Especially about feelings," she adds.

Sometimes I forget what's happening but then I'm at Walgreens and my phone number doesn't work anymore when I punch it in because it's B's phone number and it doesn't work in CVS and it doesn't work in Duane Reade and my Hulu log-in stops working and then my HBO password stops working and then I remember. The CVS and Walgreens people seem to think it is bizarre I wouldn't have a phone number to use for my purchase, but it is too long of a story to get into. Netflix kicks me out, but the *New York Times* keeps working.

"You won the lottery," Hannah says. She lives with her two toddlers' father but has a girlfriend and is on her way toward divorce. "You won the lottery because now you can have a baby with a *woman*," she says.

I know what she means. I didn't win the IVF-grant lottery but this one I won. Some people spend years trying to extricate themselves from long-term relationships. But freedom has been spoon-fed to me. The ultimate get-out-of-jail-free card. Out of wife day care.

Riley is ironing and I tell her I like her sweatpants. She irons every time we're together, in the morning, before she goes to work. We usually have the television on in the background, half watching *The Challenge.*

"What kind are they?" I ask.

"The style or the brand?"

"Brand."

"Vuori."

"Oh yeah, my ex-husband used to wear that shit."

She rolls her eyes and we laugh. When someone on a dating app asks me what kind of people I usually date I say, *lesbians who iron.* I get messages from people asking if a steamer counts.

In my new apartment a few blocks from my old one, there are a family of groundhogs in the yard and a bird's nest on the upper-left corner of the deck. I watch them in the mornings as I work. This could be the part in the book where my research of groundhogs becomes a metaphor. I would poetically write about this family of groundhogs. They'd represent something like the family I don't have and ultimately I, the narrator, would accept that I didn't have it because I had so much else. It would end with me watching the groundhogs out my window, or maybe the bird giving birth. You would close the book knowing everything would be okay. The reader would feel closure and the writer would feel closure.

One morning while writing there is a blue jay where the groundhogs usually are. Immediately I google the meaning and Google tells me what I want to hear, which is that blue jays are a good omen and that good news is coming my way.

I think about a writing workshop I'd recently led where someone had written an essay and there was a scene where she'd described talking to a seagull. Everyone in the workshop got stuck on this detail, talking about its meaning for ten minutes, until someone, frustrated, blurted out, "Sometimes a bird is just a bird!"

The summer of divorce is the most urban summer I've had since 2006, easy. When the second day of September hits, I realized I haven't gone swimming once. Haven't picked berries. Haven't been to a farmers market, haven't been on a hike. The summer of divorce is a constant pounding of pavement. I am in Paris and New York City and Hudson, on foot. I walk to the dentist. Walk to the gynecologist. Walk to the dermatologist. Walk to the Amtrak. Walk to Planned Parenthood. Walk to the post office, walk to JD's for enchiladas and to do my laundry. I don't turn on my oven. I unsubscribe from *Smitten Kitchen* and *NYT Cooking*. There aren't grocery lists in my Notes app anymore, just drafts and drafts and drafts of melodramatic break-up texts I am sending to Riley every other week. I don't shut the door all the way when I pee, and I don't make my bed unless I feel like it, and live on French presses of coffee and bread. I collect matchboxes from cocktail bars and soaps from hotels.

One morning I spend ten minutes trying to convince Riley to have sex instead of leaving the bed for work.

"You have to beg," she says.

"I *have* been begging."

"You're using too many words," she responds. "Beg with your body."

Knowing sperm is available for purchase, just knowing that it's a possibility, helps me function. A doctor once told me that she prescribes Xanax for people because even if the people don't take it they feel better knowing they have the option.

On Airbnb, I have a wish list saved called IVF Prague. It's pure comedy now, the fact that I was strongly considering doing IVF in Prague. The Google Flights alerts from JFK to Prague come through to my email.

I remember one of the mornings when we were driving to the fertility clinic for an IUI. I commented to B that he never wore his wedding ring. It was uncomfortable, he said. The dish soap got underneath it.

I'm at dinner with a friend of a friend. She says, "*You* were married to a man?"

"Yeah, who hasn't been?" I respond.

I log into my patient portal from the fertility clinic.

Blood work: twenty-six times.
IUI: three times.
Vaginal ultrasounds: six.
Prescriptions: eight.
Medications: letrozole, Ovidrel, clomiphene, Prometrium, Synthroid, letrozole again, Ovidrel again, Prometrium again.

The word "infertility" seems like such a scam. If someone is diagnosed with "unexplained infertility" and then gets pregnant a few years later, or swallows Clomid and gets pregnant with twins, or divorces one partner and becomes pregnant with another, or seven years later, does the diagnosis go away?

Most doctors only approve fertility treatments for heterosexual couples after they've tried for one year by having sex. But which doctors are checking? Unless there are cameras watching these straight couples, there's no way to prove they've tried.

It depends on the state, but it is common for queer people have to go through six rounds of failed IUIs before being diagnosed with infertility. You're only allowed to do IVF once you prove (prove!) your infertility. In more than half of European countries, IVF for queer couples and single women is banned, illegal.

If I had walked into a fertility clinic during my hetero marriage, I'd be diagnosed with infertility, and they'd recommend I go straight to IVF. If I walk into that same clinic in a queer partnership, having done three IUIs, I'd have to have three more IUIs before I would be diagnosed as infertile. My diagnosis is dependent on whom I am dating.

A woman walks into a fertility clinic . . .

In a 2019 *New Yorker* article, "The Case for Redefining Infertility," Anna Louie Sussman writes:

> Scholars, activists, and medical practitioners have begun urging policymakers to adopt a more expansive definition of infertility. They argue that infertility is only sometimes physiological; it's also possible to suffer from social infertility, a condition that stems from the broader factors that shape our lives.

Cleaning out a closet in my apartment, I find dream journals from a couple of years back that I don't remember writing.

Trying to run up a hill but turned around—too hard. There was a couple on the path and they told me I could do it but that it would be hard.

Someone got a breast reduction.

I was pregnant and people told me if you're pregnant you need to wear a turtleneck.

Cameron Diaz's boobs.

I had mail from mom and it was a book about a bisexual girl waiting for a bus.

Dream I was so relaxed that I forgot to go to my blood test.

We were cracking babies out of eggs and on the third egg we finally got one.

Dad said, "How did you think you'd get pregnant with a butch lesbian?"

Having pepperoni pizza at a bar with me, Riley asks, "What do you think you'd have ended up being if you weren't a writer?"

"Probably a barista, or working at a store full time," I said. "But writing for fun when I wasn't at work," I added.

Riley roasts me consistently for not having a job. "I have multiple jobs," I argue back. I teach writing, I write books, I work at the pants store on Saturdays.

"Yeah, you have a *career*—but you don't have a *job*," she retorts.

It makes me think of the Cheryl Strayed line, "You don't have a career. You have a life."

After pizza, we sit on my deck with Hannah and her girlfriend drinking tequila. Hannah turns to Riley and me.

"What're the top three things you guys talk about?"

"Probably the sex we've already had, the sex we're going to have, and how much the Amtrak sucks," I say, and Riley agrees, adding, "And our exes or people we've dated."

Secretly, occasionally, privately, I gloat that they were all wrong. Everyone who told me to relax and I'd get pregnant, everyone who told me to take more zinc or do acupuncture, everyone who told me, "When it happens, it happens," telling me to make a shrine, bring the baby milk, do visualization, do acupuncture, take more iron, take CoQ10. Wrong, wrong, wrong, you morons. Some delays are protection.

I remember how I used to visualize a high chair at our kitchen counter.

You were all wrong and I was right. I *knew* something was wrong, even though I wasn't right about what it was. I knew something was wrong even though I couldn't articulate it. I thought it was perhaps blocked fallopian tubes, and it ended up being sex workers in Geneva. So be it. I was still right.

Go be right then, Riley says, annoyed, when I'm having to be right, over text during one of our miscommunications, which start happening almost daily.

"Do you want to be right or do you want to be married?" married people and marriage experts like to condescendingly say. Apparently I'd rather be right!

I have lunch with a writer who is working on a piece about becoming a single mom by choice. She'd been married and half-heartedly trying to get pregnant with the man she was married to, but they divorced because she realized he wasn't the person she wanted to have a child with. She did eight IUIs and on the eighth became pregnant with her son.

She says that she followed her heart to create this life of being a mom, and now that she is a mom, she has to follow her heart less, because that's part of parenting. She says not to choose a sperm donor over six feet. She's 5'3" and so am I, and if the donor is 6'3", it will be hard to get the baby out. We sit on a patio and we both order a dish with summer corn and feta. We hug when we part. It's hard to walk away from her, from what she represents.

Riley and I are in bed on a Saturday night and when we have sex we joke about how it will get me pregnant and I come hard. One night we watch the comedian Jerrod Carmichael talk about how sometimes when he's having really good sex he feels like he will impregnate his male partner. He says, "Then I remember what kind of sex I'm having."

We fall asleep watching a show about how Cheez-Its are made after we finish watching the movie *Bound*. We fall asleep holding hands. We kiss each other's backs when we spoon. Her face looks like she's concentrating really hard and when I ask her what she's thinking about, she says, "I'm remembering."

"Remembering what?"

"The moment."

When I'm thinking about Riley, I don't have to be thinking about what happened. When I'm thinking about Riley I don't have to be thinking about fertility, about how another year has passed. I don't have to think about probiotics or prebiotics or my stepdaughter. I only have to think about the moment I'm in. I know this escapism will likely cost me something later and I'm okay with that.

I notice rope tied around the headboard of her bed.

"You never use this with me," I say.

"Nope, not with you."

One morning walking to the L train after leaving Riley's, there are tears in my eyes from being so connected and in my body. I send a voice memo to Jasmin (of the infamous "in short—I'm gay" post) and she voice memos me back saying, "Eros is literally the meaning of life, straight people have no idea what life can be like, the play and exploration of it all, the novelty of being alive."

The first time I'm supposed to have an appointment with the fertility clinic (Infertility clinic? I still never know) about doing IUIs with a sperm donor, I miss the appointment. I'm normally organized in terms of work and use multiple calendars. A whiteboard, a Google Calendar. I try to not make any meaning out of this, no easy self-deprecating jokes about how I'm not responsible enough to have a baby since I can't even remember a Zoom meeting.

I remember how B and I tried to make meaning where there wasn't any. At our first IUI, we sat in the parking lot facing a hill. We saw a bunny frolic on the hill, and we attempted to force it to be good luck. I didn't believe it and he didn't either.

Receiving a newsletter from a sperm bank you never signed up for is unsettling. You're sitting there drinking your coffee, maybe editing a student essay while also looking at bras on sale at Natori, reminding yourself to drink water, listening to Chappell Roan, and then of course you click over to your Gmail and the Seattle Sperm Bank has sent you a newsletter. What does a sperm bank newsletter even entail? you wonder, so you open it, even though that's probably bad for your algorithm. The newsletter opens with a child wearing a pink headband and pink dress riding what looks like a unicorn. The unicorn is decorated with pink flowers around its body and its horn is metallic. You figure this is a stock image—unicorns aren't real!—but underneath the photo it says, "Happy birthday to Soren," so the photo is actually real, whatever "real" means.

I have a dream that I am at my friend's house with their kids and a box of sperm shows up for me. I don't remember ordering it, but figure since it is here, I'll use it. We are all figuring it out together, but then we realize we've forgotten the most important part—no one knows how to insert the sperm into my vagina. Then I have to go to the store for something, and while I am out, my friend calls me and says we should wrap up this process since his kids have school in the morning.

I reschedule my appointment with the clinic. I think about making a list of questions for them. I'd like to ask them if they think it's possible bodies reject sperm if it isn't from the person you're supposed to raise a child with. I want to ask them how to choose a donor. I want to ask them if they think I'm acting from a place of mania. I want to ask them how to grieve. I want to ask them how I could have been so sure about my future. We don't have that kind of relationship, though.

What used to be called "single mom by choice" has evolved to "She is having a baby with herself." Or, "They are having a baby with themself." Once I start considering it, friends keep mentioning people they know who are doing it. One night I meet one outside the bar I'm in, sitting on the stoop of her apartment eating Chinese food out of a takeout container.

On the phone again with the fertility clinic's hold message: *We offer affordable and innovative ways to create your family.* This time I'm here for the innovative way. I tell the doctor I'm back but my *situation has changed.* I learn that I cannot move forward because I am still legally married and I can't do anything without a divorce decree.

When I'd learned whom I was married to, I wanted to get divorced as fast as I could. I found a website that promised it would be fast, paid $245 for it, then sent B a Venmo request. After I paid the fee and filled out the form and sent it in, I had to get something notarized. I found an online notary and felt like a tech wizard. I sent in the notarized forms. When I checked on my status a few weeks later, the ephemeral "Michael" sent back an email to all "clients" that his mother had unexpectedly died. I sent him a bereavement note, because I assumed Michael was going to be someone somewhat important in my life: He was helping me get divorced. Michael never responded.

"EZ divorce?" a friend later says to me. "Did you think it was like E-ZPass?"

The fertility clinic sends me a list of costs.

IUI Cycle Fees:
$143.00 p/ Lab
$15.00 Venipuncture
$254.10 Ultrasound
$302.50 IUI
$60.50 Sperm Thaw
$302.50 Sperm Wash [if an unwashed sample is utilized]

Amy, the doctor I speak with, talks about the cryobanks they work with: in California, Seattle, and Fairfax. She says disapprovingly that some of her clients get sperm from a place called Xytex, because it's way cheaper, I suppose. Amy clearly doesn't like Xytex and I can hear her roll her eyes.

She says something about how she knows people have to budget, "but think about what it is you're spending money on."

It is the same exact thing I say to customers at the pants store. I try to justify their purchase of almost-two-hundred-dollars-plus-tax pants because, I say, it's better than buying five pairs of crappy pants at H&M that will fall apart. They always agree with me.

My friend Shaina posts something on Instagram about looking for sperm, half joking, half serious. In their newsletter, Shaina riffs on what trans sperm could be like:

> Like maybe our sperm is like tiny little purple furry monsters with tiny little horns that aren't sharp but definitely fashionable. Maybe our sperm host little block parties and make little teeny tiny strawberry margaritas. I don't know why, but I think our sperm is femme. It definitely is.

I overhear a boy on the train ask his mom why the McDonald's workers don't go on strike. She explains what a union is. "But can't you just strike on your own?" he asks.

"That's just called quitting," she says.

"What if I run into him on the street?" I ask Riley.

"Make sure you have a lot of water balloons," she responds.

While she cracks her third beer of the morning, she says, "You're drinking *another* cup of coffee?"

She makes us grilled cheese with apple and honey and bacon before she takes the train back to the city. No one has cooked yet in my apartment. "You're meeting me at my least domestic," I say when I can't find the cheese grater, the good knife, realizing there are kitchen items I forgot to pack from my old apartment. "You're meeting me at mine," she says.

We are both living in the unknown. Riley is deciding whether to move across the country where her primary partner is, and I'm still under the fantasy of becoming a parent, thinking I'll just inseminate myself in my bed quickly. We never talk about these seismic life transitions we are in, but our time together gets heavier the hotter the summer becomes.

She sends me a song about making out by the violets. I send her a song about not being able to stop thinking about her. She sends me a song about wanting to feel my leg against her thigh. I send her a song about fucking in the morning. She sends me a song about how we are only love and longing. I send her a song about hope being a prison. She sends me a song about being in her feelings, tired, and bleeding. I send her a song about if something feels good, you should do it. She sends me a song about all the words we don't say. I send her song about kissing slowly with the lights on. She sends me a song about getting lost in the feeling, about cooking and dirty dancing in the kitchen. I send her a song about being a little in love. She sends me a song about only being as good as her mind. I send her a song that ends with fuck you. She sends me a song about being a phantom lover, about how she never learns. I send her a song about bringing out the worst in me.

We break up for the third or seventeenth time and we block each other on text, but then she Venmos me a dollar. *I don't want to lose you,* she writes under the dollar. Under the transaction I comment, *I don't want to lose you either. This is wildly painful.*

Please don't give up on me, she writes under my comment.

I'm trying not to, I say a few days later, still on Venmo.

We say we don't want to lose each other, we don't want to hurt each other, but we both do both anyway. We email, trying to work it out. I purchase a book called *The Queer Art of Failure.*

"This doesn't feel like a conversation anymore," she says.

"Just because you don't like what I'm saying doesn't make it not a conversation," I respond.

"You don't have to respond to everything I say," she comes back with.

After the breakup, I text my mom, *Too much sorrow, all the time,* not even knowing myself which loss I am referring to.

I think about a line from Maggie Millner's *Couplets*: "OK, so nothing lasts, the proof of life is the aching."

I date someone else, because though it is not a *year of yes*, it is a *summer of sure*. She is divorced with an eleven-year-old. We meet near a park bench and walk to Hall des Lumières. In advance, over text, she asks me to wear sneakers so I won't be taller than she is. She asks for consent when she touches my back through the hole in my dress. After the exhibit, we get coffee and go into a romance bookstore.

She texts later, *I was so nervous to kiss you.*

Really?

I was waiting for there not to be a Ricola cough drop in your mouth. I thought the moment would never come. Really regretted getting you that bag of them.

The first time I sleep over on her Murphy bed she makes a quinoa-and-kale salad for dinner and has my favorite candy, Good & Plenty, stocked. She puts on the movie *Pitch Perfect*, saying not to judge her for liking it, and we have sex while the movie plays, a choice I find so bizarre that I don't go to her place again. We wake up at seven in the morning and take the subway to a meditation class that begins at eight. She carries my heavy bag as we walk. She's a gym rat and has been "training for this," she says.

She says it is impossible for her to have sex without thinking and wishing she could get someone pregnant. "If we were straight we'd probably have a baby in six months," she says.

One afternoon I text her, *How many times did you and your ex-wife do IVF?* She says she thinks it was eight rounds. *It was an emotional time,* she says. Seems like an understatement.

It's wild she doesn't know the exact number. I don't think I'd ever forget it. Then again, I don't remember what exact months my IUIs were, and sometimes I can't remember if I'd done three or four or two.

Eight rounds!! I respond. *You gave it a really good shot,* I want to say, the way I've said to customers at the boutique.

I cannot imagine a world where I would do eight rounds of IVF. I couldn't imagine the world I'm currently in, either.

On a wall in Paris, I see graffiti: *We will come together again, I promise* in black paint.

A couple comes into the shop and the woman tries on multiple jump-suits. She doesn't love any of them and neither does her partner. As they're putting their coats on I hear him say to her, "You're trying on clothes you would wear before the baby, so they aren't working the same way now."

I'm sort of disarmed by this. He isn't playing the scripted game. He's actually saying what is true. She agrees and says something neutral about postpartum and her body. I can't tell if her feelings are hurt by what he said, or if she, too, is relieved because he's in reality.

My friend says that her friend has a code so I can scroll through pro-files at the sperm bank for free and that she will give me the code. It's like the old days when getting someone's HBO password was a God-given gift.

Seattle Sperm Bank sends me another newsletter. This one says you can get one vial of sperm, one free. *BOGO sale!* We don't do BOGO sales at the pants store. We're way too classy for that.

Star of Bethlehem: Neutralize Grief is a tincture I have in my kitchen. I bought it three years ago as a gift for B when his dad died. But it's me who uses it.

Mary Karr has a writing rule in her book *The Art of Memoir* warning against writing about your divorce. "Nobody sounds good writing about their divorce, let's face it," she says.

Luckily for me, I've never cared about writing rules. And I don't care about sounding good.

I ask my editor to find places where I have blind spots or sound bitter. She cuts one line, but says that otherwise blind spots and bitterness aren't my style, which is true, though my entire marriage seems to have been a blind spot.

I recall a conversation I'd had with B in the early days of the pandemic when conceiving wasn't happening as quickly as I'd wanted it to. We were walking with coffee. I'd asked him if he was open to adoption, something I'd felt suited me. As a kid and teenager I'd often fantasized about adopting a child. I'd always been interested in non-biological bonds and adored being a stepmom. My husband said it wasn't for him. I remember walking back to our apartment, deflated.

In an article in *Rolling Stone* about Shakira's divorce she said she was told to tone down her lyrics about her partner who cheated. Shakira describes when she was partnered, her life and career became more "muted" and she didn't realize until she left parts of herself she'd neglected, given up, repressed.

I purchase a book called *A Life of One's Own* by Joanna Biggs. Somewhere I hear about another book called *A Space of One's Own*.

A room of one's own.

A divorce of one's own.

A book of one's own.

Other women have similar stories to mine. Prostitutes and cocaine. It's not uncommon.

I almost left out more specifics to protect B more. In a previous memoir I'd left out his struggles with massage parlor and substance abuse addictions. My editor and I had a phone call about it. I remember standing in my leaking writing closet during our conversation, talking about making myself "the bad guy" in the book. When it was published, reviewers mentioned how patient, how perfect, he was, and seemed.

The job of a writer, particularly in nonfiction, is to be as emotionally honest as possible, as uncomfortable as that may be, and he'd let me write and publish an entire book while I was living under deceit.

But there's always another book to be written.

I notice that I've developed a physical aversion to sperm. The idea of it, the word, the thought of bringing some unknown person into my life, into my body.

Hannah gives me the book *The Carrying* by Ada Limón. I read: "What if, instead of carrying / a child, I am supposed to carry grief?"

God I hope not, I think.

Though it's already happening.

The next person I date stops mid-makeout to say, "I don't want to be in your books."

I tell a friend about it the next day.

LMAO, you're Taylor Swift, she texts.

I receive an email from the makeup brand Tarte, wishing me a happy half birthday. "Party Like It's Your Birthday," they say. "Did you know it's your half-birthday?" they say. "Yep, that's a thing," they say.

It's funny they think I don't know about my half birthday. It's funny they think I want a discount for a brand I've never used. It's funny they email me at all.

Mia and I walk around after seeing comedy at the Bell House in Brooklyn. On a cement wall, someone has written, Notice how hard you tried. I ask Mia if I can take her photo in front of the sign. I take some with her in front and some of the sign alone. She doesn't offer to take a photo of me and I don't ask her to.

It's been about three years of working at the pants store when I decide it's time to move on. As soon as I make the decision I begin to see the shop in a different light. I notice the way the sun floods through in the afternoon. The person who works on Sundays texts me: *Can we talk about how great the new vacuum is?*

I count how many pairs of life-changing pants I've purchased for myself: black, terra-cotta, rust, dark denim, light denim, pinstripe, moss. I'd thought I'd grow out of them when I got pregnant, but they all still fit me.

As for jumpsuits and overalls, I've acquired fifteen.

Before I leave the shop, I train the person replacing me. I instruct her to try on the clothes so she's able to talk about them more easily to the customers.

She tries on the pants that I tell her I like the least.

"I like unflattering pants," she says.

She's much younger than I am, so she can afford to like them.

I look into adoption again. Most people yell, "It's so expensive!" when you talk about adoption. But people spend money on all sorts of shit I never have: MFAs, regular college, fancy weddings, cars, IVF, houses, renovations. All of these American dream pursuits I haven't pursued, because I pursued writing in earnest.

The date who asked me to not put her in my books asks me to accompany her to a clinic in Manhattan that works with LGBTQ+ family planning. On the subway ride uptown, the person across from us is reading *The Montessori Baby*.

The clinic is like the ones we see in movies, nothing like the one I've been to upstate. The waiting room is full of couples and almost every chair is taken. They have a free coffee machine offering lattes, hot chocolate. There are three jars of candy, one holding Hershey's Kisses, another with Rolos, and the other with some hard pink candy. She is experiencing her first dildo cam and I give her tips, like the one about keeping her socks on for comfort. While she has her appointment, I sit in the waiting room where I can't help but notice the music targeted to my age group. They play, "If You Had My Love" by JLo, and "Heartbreaker" by Mariah Carey.

Afterward, we eat soup and salad at Le Pain Quotidien. We agree that the dildo cam is smaller than a dildo. Then we walk to Babeland and look at all the different sizes and colors of dildos.

There are some rumors going around that I've healed too quickly. Some friends think it; my mom thinks it. My mom is the only one who has the courage to say it to my face. It's funny that people think they know my healing process. It's funny that people think because I'm dating or fucking or traveling or working that I think I'm healed. It's funny that people think I don't think I'll be healing forever.

The day I'm supposed to go to the fertility or infertility clinic to do all the tests again, more saline fluid up my fallopian tubes, more dildo cams, more needles in the arm—I physically can't go. There's a block. I realize I don't think I can go there ever again.

I walk by the pants store and see instead of the handwritten chalkboard LIFE CHANGING PANTS sign there is now a digitized sign. Legit. Permanent. In addition to life-changing pants they also now offer life-changing jeans.

On the subway, I sit across from a woman with unshaven legs eating a plain container of yogurt and reading *When Things Fall Apart*.

After a thunderstorm in New York City, I'm taking an Uber to Moynihan Train Hall. The driver is chatty and warm. We drive through Times Square and she says she has never walked down Forty-Second Street but drives through it most days.

"Now it's just a normal street to me," she says.

"You're desensitized to it," I say.

Even though the ride is only about ten minutes, I learn a lot about her. I'm not asking questions but it feels organic the way she gives me information. She's in school full time, drives for Uber on weekends, is twenty-one, and had her daughter at eighteen. She says it changed her life, and though her husband tries to help, it's not enough, and when he does, she either feels he isn't doing it right, or she misses her daughter. Guilt, she says, as a full sentence. She says it wasn't planned. She says she loves her daughter so much but it is so hard. She has no time. She says more, and I'm so deeply grateful she does not ask me if I have children.

"You seem like you're doing really well with it all," I say. A weak, but true, sentiment. "I try," she responds, before dropping me off at Moynihan Train Hall. We tell each other bye, to have a good day, to stay safe, to drive safely, to stay dry. That's what we say, but we mean something else, we mean something more.

The next person I date is a photographer who says, *Aries are fun, they're entertaining.* She asks me if I always knew I wanted to be a writer; she knew she wanted to be an artist when she was ten. She has a child with her partner. They both had nonnegotiables when they met; her partner wanted a child and she wanted to be nonmonogamous and continue to travel for passion, pleasure, and work. They used her egg, donor sperm, and her partner's body to carry. She tells me she and her partner have an "exit plan" in writing with logistical and financial and parental agreements.

An exit plan! What a concept.

"What does your tattoo say?" I ask, touching her collarbone. "Young and restless?"

She laughs. It says, *Young at heart.*

"What does your necklace say, *Crying* or *Trying*?" she asks about the gold nameplate I'm wearing. I'd bought it at the pants store, because they now sell them and other necklaces that say *Enough*, *ADHD*, and *Canceled*.

"It says, *Trying*," I tell her.

I find another dream journal that I don't remember keeping from when I was married. My scribbles have predicted all of this—that B was leaving me on an island, that B was cheating with a babysitter who wore a white dress, that B was doing Adderall and binge drinking. It even said I'd run into a certain writer on the streets of Brooklyn, and a year later, I did.

"All my dreams come true," I say to people, referring to the dream journal.

One morning I wake up and the thought *I love writing* pops into my head.

My friend tells me writing is my primary partner. It's been my longest relationship, they say. Some people say God is a woman, but I think God is a writer.

One thing I know is that I trust the body, intuition, writing, in ways I did not when I began this book.

Endings are important, I tell my students. Endings and beginnings. You want the ending of your book to mimic life, to not be tied up in a bow. You want your endings and beginnings to be in conversation with each other, I say. Sometimes we swap the ending line and beginning line of the book, recreationally. It shows the writer how much power they actually have.

In Los Angeles for a book event, I walk into a shop and try on clothes for something to do. In the dressing room there is a pair of pants with a sign that reads, TRY ME! CUSTOMER FAVORITE. I try them on. They're comfortable and flattering. I don't purchase them, but the next day I go back and do. It's a fantastic marketing scheme. When I pay for them, I tell the salesperson how smart it is. She says they sell almost twenty pairs a day.

Upstate, I walk by a child in a stroller pushed by his dad. The kid's mom must be behind me on the sidewalk, and he is saying, "Mama Mama Mama."

When I get back to my apartment where only I and the groundhogs live, I sit outside where I feel the sun on my back.

In the morning, out the window my writing desk faces, for the first time, there's a fox.

This entire book—including the dedication and the following acknowledgments—was written while my father was fully alive. I'd emailed him a PDF of the book (which I don't know if he read, as his eyesight and memory had both faded) and I saw he posted the cover to his Facebook page, telling people to buy the book. I had texted him a photo of the dedication to him and he responded saying he loved it. He passed away on December 21, 2024, the evening before his seventy-fourth birthday. We'd texted that same morning. Galleys of *Trying* were being printed.

My dad was my person. He understood and saw me on a level I know many are not so fortunate to experience. He read all my books, even sold them at his music shop, supported my writing from day one. I lived with him into my late twenties, when I not only didn't make money from writing but lost money from writing. He told me, "You get good at what you do, so if you look at your phone, you get really good at looking at your phone. If you write, you get really good at writing."

I love you Dad, and I miss you all day every day.

This one was for you. And I think you knew that.

In loving memory
Robert D. Caldwell
1950–2024

Acknowledgments

Thank you: JD Urban, Marty Geren, Siena, Hannah Tennant-Moore, Mia Arias Tsang, Alex Alberto, Noelle Bruneau, Divna Encheva, LA Warman, and Jasmin Sandelson. Your friendship kept me functioning. Yuka Igarashi: Thank you for asking the questions that needed to be asked, meeting me in my process, your patience, sharing my brain, letting me write chaos in real time, and helping the book emerge however it needed to. I don't know anyone else as radically creative. I'm going to miss working on this book with you. Thank you: LDMK. <3 As usual, you were right—you will always be with me, and me with you. Everyone at Graywolf: Marisa Atkinson, Katie Dublinski, Carmen Giménez, Claire Laine, Ethan Nosowsky, Casey O'Neil, Veronica Silva, and the entire wolf pack, thank you for taking risks on strange books like this one and all the books you've been publishing that I've been reading for fifteen years. I feel extremely lucky. Thank you to the one agent who gets it: Rebecca Gradinger at United Talent Agency. When I first told you about this project, you called it "an art-monster book." You weren't wrong. Thank you, Laurie-Maude Chenard at United Talent Agency. Thank you to the GGC and GGC Paris. Thank you, Core Four: Jillian Eugenios, Emily J. Smith, and Courtney (coco) Priess. Thank you to Danielle Ribner at Loup, for the job, for your friendship, and for keeping me stocked in life-changing clothing. Thank you, Elizabeth Ellen and Chelsea Martin, for reading the first twenty pages many years ago. Thank you to my mom who read a draft and wrote notes for me. Thank you to my dad for his great one-liners. I won the lottery in the parent department. My students in my yearlong classes and queer-breakup class and all other classes, retreats, and mentorships: You give me so much. You're all over this book. Thank you to indie booksellers, libraries, and readers. You've helped me create a life of writing.

CHLOÉ CALDWELL is the author of the novella *Women*, the memoir *The Red Zone*, and the essay collections *I'll Tell You in Person* and *Legs Get Led Astray*. Her essays have appeared in the *New York Times*, *Vogue*, *Bon Appétit*, the *Cut*, MSNBC, *Autostraddle*, *Longreads*, and *Nylon* and in anthologies including *Goodbye to All That: Writers on Loving and Leaving New York* and *Without a Net: The Female Experience of Growing Up Working Class* and *Sluts*. She offers writing support at scrappyliterary.com. Caldwell lives in Hudson, New York.

Instagram: @ChloeeeeCaldwell

Website: www.chloesimonne.com

Graywolf Press publishes risk-taking, visionary writers who transform culture through literature. As a nonprofit organization, Graywolf relies on the generous support of its donors to bring books like this one into the world.

This publication is made possible, in part, by the voters of Minnesota through a Minnesota State Arts Board Operating Support grant, thanks to a legislative appropriation from the arts and cultural heritage fund. Significant support has also been provided by the National Endowment for the Arts and other generous contributions from foundations, corporations, and individuals. To these supporters we offer our heartfelt thanks.

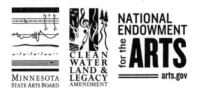

To learn more about Graywolf's books and authors or make a tax-deductible donation, please visit www.graywolfpress.org.

The text of *Trying* is set in Perpetua MT Pro.
Book design by Rachel Holscher.
Composition by Bookmobile Design & Digital
Publisher Services, Minneapolis, Minnesota.
Manufactured by Friesens on acid-free,
100 percent postconsumer wastepaper.